Clinical trials in psychiatry

Brian S. Everitt
*Professor of Behavioural Statistics,
Institute of Psychiatry, King's College,
London, UK*

and

Simon Wessely
*Department of Psychological medicine, GKT
School of Medicine and Institute of Psychiatry,
London, UK*

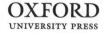
OXFORD
UNIVERSITY PRESS

OXFORD
UNIVERSITY PRESS

Great Clarendon Street, Oxford OX2 6DP

Oxford University Press is a department of the University of Oxford.
It furthers the University's objective of excellence in research,
scholarship, and education by publishing worldwide in

Oxford New York

Auckland Bangkok Buenos Aires Cape Town Chennai
Dar es Salaam Delhi Hong Kong Istanbul Karachi Kolkata
Kuala Lumpur Madrid Melbourne Mexico City Mumbai Nairobi
Sao Paulo Shanghai Taipei Tokyo Toronto

Oxford is a registered trade mark of Oxford University Press
in the UK and in certain other countries

Published in the United States
by Oxford University Press Inc., New York

British Library Cataloguing in Publication Data

Data available

ISBN 0 19 852642 3

10 9 8 7 6 5 4 3 2 1

Typeset by Integra Software Services Pvt. Ltd, Pondicherry, India
Printed in Great Britain
on acid-free paper by Biddles Ltd., Guildford & King's Lynn.

Preface

Estimates of the annual cost of mental health problems to the United Kingdom range from £7bn to £32bn; mental health accounts for a quarter of all GP consultations. Given these figures it is not surprising that the search for effective treatments in psychiatry continues apace. From new drug therapies for schizophrenia to the use of cognitive behaviour therapy in managing depression, psychiatric research workers remain committed to discovering the best means of overcoming the misery that is mental illness. But for progress to be maintained and hopefully accelerated, competing treatments need to be assessed and compared in the most rigorous manner available. Such rigour is provided by the randomised clinical trial, which as implemented in psychiatry, is the subject of this book. We hope the material included will be useful for trainee psychiatrists who are very likely to be involved in clinical trials at some time in their careers, for psychiatrists currently applying clinical trial methodology and for other researchers in mental health who need to assess the implications of the results from psychiatric trials for patient care.

We would like to thank the following people who have provided ideas, suggestions, criticisms and often all three, during the preparation of this book; Anders Skrondal, Catherine Gilvarry, Clive Adams, Sir Iain Chalmers, Barbara Farrell, Matthew Hotopf and Mike Slade.

Finally thanks are due to Harriet Meteyard for much help during the writing of the book, particularly with the references.

London
March 2003

B.S.E
S.W

Contents

Chapter 1

Treatments, good, bad or worthless—and how do we tell?

1.1 Treatments worthless—and worse

All who drink of this remedy recover in a short time, except those whom it does not help, who all die. Therefore, it is obvious that it fails only in incurable cases.

This aphorism is generally attributed to Galen (AD 130–200), a Greek physician, who was destined to dominate medicine for many centuries and who wrote with such conviction and dogmatism that few doctors dared to criticize him. He was a prodigious writer and in one of his many books he gives an account of his own parents, describing his father as amiable, just and benevolent, and his mother as thoroughly objectionable, a woman who was always shouting at her husband and displaying her evil temper by biting her serving-maids. His father had a dream that his son was destined one day to become a great physician and this encouraged him to send Galen to Pergamos and to Smyrna for a preliminary grounding in philosophy, and then onto Alexandria to specialize in medicine.

The veneration of dogma proclaimed by Galen and other authoritative people largely stifled any interest in experimentation or proper scientific exploration in medicine until well into the seventeenth century. Even the few who did attempt to increase their knowledge by close observation or simple experiment often interpreted their findings in the light of the currently accepted dogma. When, for example, Andreas Vesalius, a sixteenth century Belgian physician, first dissected a human heart and did not find 'pores', said by Galen to perforate the septum separating the ventricular chambers, the Belgian assumed the openings were invisible to the eye. It was only several years after his initial investigation that Vesalius had the confidence to declare that 'pores' did not exist.

Similarly the announcement of the discovery of the circulation of the blood by an English physician, William Harvey, in 1628, met with violent opposition, since it contradicted Galen's view that blood flowed to and fro in a tide-like movement within arteries and veins. Even when it was admitted rather grudgingly that Harvey was probably correct, a defender of the established view wrote that if the new findings did not agree with Galen, the discrepancy should be attributed to the fact that nature had changed; one should not admit that the master had been wrong!

For the medieval physician, choice of treatment depended largely on the results of observing one or two patients or on reports from colleagues, again usually based on very limited numbers of observations. But since patients rather inconveniently vary in their responses to treatment, this was often the recipe for the development of treatments that were disastrously ineffective when applied more generally. Each proposed treatment (however absurd) might be taken up by enthusiasts only to be dropped when another (often equally absurd) became fashionable. Even the oath taken by Western physicians since the time of Hippocrates, in which they swear to protect their patients 'from whatever is deleterious and mischievous', has not managed to stop many assaultive therapies being given or to lessen the persistence of barbarous practices like copious blood-letting. Even the most powerful members of society were vulnerable to the ill-informed, if well-intentioned physician. At 8 o'clock on Monday morning of 2 February 1685, for example, King Charles II of England was being shaved in his bedroom. With a sudden cry he fell backward and had a violent convulsion.

He became unconscious, rallied once or twice, and after a few days, died. Doctor Scarburgh, one of the twelve or fourteen physicians called to treat the stricken king, recorded the efforts made to cure the patient.

As the first step in treatment the king was bled to the extent of a pint from a vein in his right arm. Next his shoulder was cut into and the incised area was 'cupped' to suck out an additional eight ounces of blood. After this, the drugging began. An emetic and purgative were administered, and soon after a second purgative. This was followed by an enema containing antimony, sacred bitters, rock salt, mallow leaves, violets, beetroot, camomile flowers, fennel seed, linseed, cinnamon, cardamom seed, saphron, cochineal, and aloes. The enema was repeated in two hours and a purgative given. The king's head was shaved and a blister raised on his scalp. A sneezing powder of hellebore root was administered and also a powder of cowslip flowers 'to strengthen his brain.' The cathartics were repeated at frequent intervals and interspersed with a soothing drink composed of barley water, liquorice, and sweet almond. Likewise white wine, absinthe, and anise were given, as also were extracts of thistle leaves, mint, rue, and angelica. For external treatment a plaster of Burgundy pitch and pigeon dung was applied to the king's feet. The bleeding and purging continued, and to the medicaments were added melon seeds, manna, slippery elm, black cherry water, an extract of flowers of lime, lily of the valley, peony, lavender, and dissolved pearls. Later came gentian root, nutmeg, quinine and cloves. The king's condition did not improve, indeed it grew worse, and in the emergency forty drops of extract of human skull were administered to allay convulsions. A rallying dose of Raleigh's antidote was forced down the king's throat; this antidote contained an enormous number of herbs and animal extracts. Finally bezoar stone was given. 'Then', said Scarburgh, 'Alas! After an ill-fated night his serene majesty's strength seemed exhausted to such a degree that the whole assembly of physicians lost all hope and became despondent; still so as not to appear to fail in doing their duty in any detail, they brought into play the most active cordial'.

As a sort of grand summary to this pharmaceutical debauch, a mixture of Raleigh's antidote, pearl julep, and ammonia was forced down the throat of the dying king.

Occasionally serendipitous observations led to more suitable treatments being discovered. An example is provided by the Renaissance surgeon, Ambroise Pare, when treating wounds suffered by soldiers during the battle to capture the castle of Villaine in 1537. Pare intended to apply the standard treatment of pouring boiled oil over the wound but ran out of oil. He then substituted a digestive made of egg yolks, oil of roses, and turpentine. The superiority of the new treatment became evident the day after the battle:

> I raised myself very early to visit them, when beyond my hope I found those to whom I applied the digestive medicament feeling but little pain, their wounds neither swollen nor inflamed, and having slept through the night. The others to whom I had applied the boiling oil were feverish with much pain and swelling about their wounds. Then I determined never again to burn thus so cruelly by arquebusses.

By the late seventeenth and early eighteenth century some scientists and physicians began to adopt a more sceptical attitude to the pronouncements of authoritative figures and medicine began a slow march from dogmatic, even mystical, certainty to proper scientific uncertainty. One of the most notable examples illustrating this change is provided by James Lind's investigation into the treatment of scurvy.

Scurvy is a disease characterized by debility, blood changes, spongy gums, and hemorrhages in the tissues of the body. The symptoms come on gradually with failure of strength and mental depression. Then follow sallow complexion, sunken eyes, tender gums, and muscular pains. These symptoms may continue for weeks, gradually worsening. Teeth fall out and hemorrhages, often massive, penetrate muscles and other tissues. The last stages of scurvy are marked by profound exhaustion, fainting and complications such as diarrhea and pulmonary or kidney troubles, any of which may bring about death. In 1932 it was discovered that the cause of scurvy is deficiency of vitamin C, and even in desperate cases, recovery may be anticipated when the deficient vitamin is supplied, by injection or orally.

But three hundred years ago physicians knew only that scurvy was common, was often fatal, and was a severe problem for mariners, causing more deaths in wartime than did the enemy. It is, for example, recorded that in 1740, Lord Anson took six ships on a world cruise and lost some 1200 of his men to the disease. There was some speculation that scurvy and diet were connected but it was Lind who first investigated the relationship in a proper scientific fashion.

James Lind was a Scottish physician who took his MD degree at Edinburgh in 1748 and was physician at the Haslar hospital for men of the Royal Navy, Gosport, Hampshire, England from 1758 until his death. In his book, *A Treatise on the Scurvy*, published in 1754, he gives the following description of his landmark study:

> On the 20th May 1747, I took twelve patients in the scurvy, on board the Salisbury at sea. Their cases were as similar as I could have them. They all in general had putrid gums, the spots and lassitude, with weakness of their knees. They lay together in one

place, being a proper apartment for the sick in the forehold; and had one diet in common to all, viz. water-gruel sweetened with sugar in the morning; fresh mutton broth often times for dinner; at other times puddings, boiled biscuit with sugar etc. And for supper, barley and raisins, rice and currants, sago and wine, or the like. Two of these were ordered each a quart of cider a day. Two others took twenty-five gutts of elixir vitriol three times a day, upon an empty stomach; using a gargle strongly acidulated with it for their mouths. Two others took two spoonfuls of vinegar three times a day, upon an empty stomach: having their gruels and their other food well acidulated with it, as also the gargle for their mouths. Two of the worst patients, with the tendons in the ham rigid (a symptom none of the rest had) were put under a course of sea-water. Of this they drank half a pint every day, and sometimes more or less as it operated, by way of a gentle physic. Two others had each two oranges and one lemon given them every day. These they eat with greediness, at different times, upon an empty stomach. They continued but six days under this course, having consumed the quantity that could be spared. The two remaining patients, took the bigness of a nutmeg three times a day of an electuary recommended by a hospital-surgeon, made of garlic, mustard-feed, rad, raphan, balsam of Peru, and gum myrr; using for common drink barley water well acidulated with tamarinds; by a decoction of which, with the addition of cremor tartar, they were greatly purged three or four times during the course. The consequence was, that the most sudden and visible good effects were perceived from the use of the oranges and lemons; one of those who had taken them, being at the end of six days fit for duty. The spots were not indeed at that time quite off his body, nor his gums sound; but without any other medicine, than a gargle of elixir vitriol, he became quite healthy before we came into Plymouth, which was on the 16th June. The other was the best recovered of any in his condition; and being now deemed pretty well, was appointed nurse to the rest of the sick.

In spite of the relative clear-cut nature of his findings, Lind still advised that the best treatment for scurvy involved placing stricken patients in 'pure dry air'. No doubt the reluctance to accept oranges and lemons as treatment for the disease had something to do with their expense compared to the 'dry air' treatment. In fact it was a further 40 years before Gilbert Blane, Commissioner of the Board of the Care of Sick and Wounded Seamen, succeeded in persuading the Admiralty to make the use of lemon juice compulsory in the British Navy. But once again the question of cost quickly became an issue with limes, which were cheaper, being substituted for lemons. Economy thus condemned the British sailor to be referred to for the next two hundred years as 'limeys'.

The characteristics of Lind's investigation which make it so notable for the time are its *comparison* of different treatments and the similarity of the patients at the commencement of the study, i.e. they were all at a similar stage of the illness and were all on a similar diet. As we shall see in the next chapter these characteristics are much like those demanded in a modern clinical trial.

But Lind's systematic approach to treatment evaluation was, in the eighteenth century, the exception rather than the rule, and personal observation was still highly regarded by most clinicians as the most appropriate way of providing suitable procedures for alleviating the suffering of their patients. The result was the continuation of such 'treatments' as blood-letting, purging, complicated diets and even starvation. It was not until the beginning of the nineteenth century that a few courageous physicians acknowledged that personal observations on a small number of patients, however acutely made, are unlikely to tell the whole story, and pronounced that most treatments then in use were essentially worthless. Pierre-Charles-Alexander Louis, for example, became famous for rejecting the established doctrine of blood-letting as a medical treatment. Through observation he showed that slightly more people who were bled died than people who were not. Clinicians were increasingly forced to admit that the cupboard of specific remedies was virtually bare, and so concentrated their efforts on accurate diagnosis and prognosis rather than treatment. During the next hundred years or so *some* progress was made in identifying effective treatments for particular conditions, for example, the heart drug digoxin from the foxglove and aspirin from the bark of the willow tree. But the real therapeutic revolution has occurred in the last 75 years or so and has seen the introduction of effective treatments for a vast range of diseases. The reasons behind this revolution involve a complex mixture of progress in pharmacology and medical technology well described in Le Fanu (1999). But as more and more potential treatments were developed, the need grew for some scientifically acceptable form of procedure by which their advantages and disadvantages could be assessed. Fortunately this need was met in the 1930s/1940s by the introduction of the *controlled clinical trial*, the story of which we take up in Chapter 2. Here we move on to say a little more about treatments specific to that branch of medicine with which this book is largely concerned, namely *psychiatry*.

1.2   A brief history of treating the mentally ill

> The mentally ill have always been with us—to be feared, marvelled at, laughed at, pitied or tortured, but all too seldom cured.
>
> Alexander and Selesnick, *The History of Psychiatry*, 1967.

In his dictionary of Psychology, the late Professor Stuart Sutherland defines psychiatry as 'the medical speciality that deals with mental disorders'. An almost equally brief definition appears in Campbell's Psychiatric Dictionary, namely, 'the medical speciality concerned with the study, diagnosis, treatment and prevention of behaviour disorders'. In terms of either definition it would appear that psychiatry has a long history; Pythagoreans, for example, employed a form of music therapy with emotionally ill patients (see Gordon, 1949), and Aretaeus (AD 50–130) observed mentally ill patients and did careful follow-up studies on them. As a result, he established that manic and depressive states often occur in the same individual and that lucid intervals generally exist between manic and depressive periods.

But a thousand years on such a seemingly enlightened approach to the mentally ill had been largely abandoned in favour of viewing the insane as wild beasts who should be kept constantly in fetters. Indeed according to Foucault (1961), 'madness borrowed its face from the mask of the beast'. In early medieval times beating, incarceration and restraint were the 'treatments' endured by the majority of the mentally ill. Insanity was almost universally regarded as a spiritual trial which one had to undergo as a punishment for vice, a test of faith, or a method of purging sin—a form of Purgatory on Earth—which could be dealt with only by spiritual remedies such as exorcism or being locked up in a church overnight. Gradually other approaches to treatment were introduced although most were equally harsh; bleeding, vomiting, and purging for mentally ill patients were common, as were more whimsical forms of treatment such as whirling or spinning a madman round on a pivot. These treatments were in addition to the continued use of manacles and chains for restraint. Apart from their harshness, what these treatments also had in common was that they were almost universally ineffective.

It was not until the seventeenth century that the tide of opinion seemed to have turned against rough treatment. For example, on 18 July 1646 the Court of Governors of Bethlem Hospital ordered 'that no officer or servant shall give any blows or ill language to any of the mad folks on pain of loosing his place' and at the same hospital in 1677 the Governors propounded a rule that 'No Officer or Servant shall beat or abuse any Lunatik, nor offer any force to them, but upon absolute, Necessity, for the better governing of them'. As a substitute for coercion, some institutes housing the insane began to offer kindness, attention to health, cleanliness and comfort. Reformers such as John Monro pioneered the introduction of 'moral treatment' which stressed the value of occupation to combat the dangers of idleness, and the need for patients to be dealt with tenderly and with affection. Such an approach was now considered to be more likely to restore reason than harshness or severity.

But although there was an increasing desire for caring to replace constraint in dealing with the mentally disturbed, drugs such as corium, digitalis, antimony, and chloral were still used to quieten disruptive patients, replacing physical fetters with pharmacological ones. And despite the best efforts of the advocates of the moral treatment approach, asylums housing the insane often remained depressing and degrading places until well into the twentieth century, as is illustrated by the following account of a visit by a newly appointed psychiatrist in 1953 to the chronic ward of a mental hospital in Cambridge in the United Kingdom (given in Le Fanu, 1999):

> I was taken in by someone who had a key to unlock the door and lock it behind you. The crashing of keys in the lock was an essential part of asylum life then just as it is today in jail. This led into a big bare room, overcrowded with people, with scrubbed floors, bare wooden tables, benches screwed to the floor, people milling around in shapeless clothing. There was a smell in the air of urine, paraldehyde, floor polish, boiled cabbage and carbolic soap—the asylum smell. Some wards were full of tousled, apathetic people just sitting in a row because for twenty years the nurses had been saying 'sit down, shut up'. Others were noisy. At the back of the ward were the padded cells, in which would be one or two patients, smeared with faeces, shouting obscenities at anybody who came near. A scene of human degradation.

Sadly many early twentieth century treatments for the mentally ill patient appear in retrospect equally as harsh as those used centuries earlier, and in the main, almost equally ineffective in producing a cure. One positive change from earlier times, however, was that now some clinicians began to take the first small steps to evaluating treatments scientifically by making qualitative and quantitative observations and measurements. Empiricism was, at last, about to play a role in psychiatric practice. Both the harshness of treatment and the attempt at a more scientific approach to evaluation can be illustrated in the context of the theory relating focal infection to mental disorders proposed by Dr Henry A. Cotton in the 1920s. According to Dr Cotton:

> The so called functional psychoses we believe today to be due to a combination of many factors, but the most constant one is the intra-cerebral, bio-chemical cellular disturbance arising from circulating toxins originating in chronic foci of infection, situated anywhere in the body, associated probably with secondary disturbance of the endocrin system. Instead of considering the psychosis as a disease entity, it should be considered as a symptom, and often a terminal symptom of a long continued masked infection, the toxaemia of which acts directly on the brain.

Dr Cotton identified that infection of the teeth and tonsils are the most important foci to be considered, but the stomach and in female patients, the cervix could also be sources of infection responsible, according to Dr Cotton's theory for the mental condition of the patient. The logical treatment for the mentally ill resulting from Dr Cotton's theory was surgical elimination of the chronically infected tissue, all infected teeth and tonsils certainly and for many patients, colectomies. Additionally female patients might require enucleation of the cervix, or in some cases complete removal of fallopian tubes and ovaries. Such treatment was, according to Dr Cotton, enormously successful with out of 1400 patients treated only 42 needing to remain in hospital.

The focal infection theory of functional psychoses was not universally accepted, neither were the striking results said to have been obtained by the removal of these infections. So in 1922, Drs Kopeloff and Cheney of the New York State Psychiatric Institute undertook a study to investigate Dr Cotton's proposed treatment in the spirit of, in their own words:

> an approach free from prejudice and without preconceived ideas as to the possible results

To achieve this laudable if somewhat pious aim, Kopeloff and Cheney planned their study in the form of an experiment. All the patients were divided into two groups as nearly identical as possible. All members of one group received operative treatment for foci of infection in teeth and tonsils, while members of the other group received no such treatment and consequently could be regarded as controls. No doubt Kepeloff and Cheney's study would have been hard pressed to have gained ethical approval today, but despite its ethical and probable scientific limitations it did produce results (summarized here in Table 1.1) that cast grave doubts over removal of focal infections as a treatment for some types of mental illness, and indirectly at least, drove a nail into the coffin of Dr Cotton's theory as to the cause of these conditions.

Dr Cotton's suggested treatment for patients with functional psychoses was severe, but not more so than other 'physical therapies' which became popular in the 1930s and 1940s. Insulin coma, for example, required patients to be given large

Table 1.1 Results from Kopeloff and Cheney's study.

	Demential praecox		Manic depressive	
	Controls	Operated	Controls	Operated
Number of cases	15	17	15	9
Recovered	—	—	5	4
Improved	5	5	8	1
Total benefited	5	5	13	5
Unimproved	10	12	2	4
Left Hospital	3	5	6	3

doses of insulin which, by lowering the blood sugar, induced a comatose state from which they would be rescued by a large dose of glucose (if they were amongst the lucky ones—some patients died). According to Sargant and Slater (1944), 'reliable statistics are mostly in favour of the treatment', although this claim needs to considered along side their recommendation as to how to select patients for treatment:

> It is rarely indeed that facilities will exist for the treatment by a full course of insulin of all schizophrenics coming under observation, and it is therefore important not to waste the treatment on patients not very likely to respond while denying it to the favourable cases.

Perhaps the most severe of the physical therapies was a lobotomy where the brain was cut with a knife. The operation was pioneered by Egas Moniz, a Lisbon neurologist, and later taken up enthusiastically by psychiatrists such as William Sargant of St Thomas's Hospital in the United Kingdom. Evaluation of the effectiveness of the therapy was largely anecdotal, and even an enthusiast such as Sargant knew that the operation was often performed at a price:

> It is probable that the highest powers of the intellect are affected detrimentally, and if the patient shows little sign of this in his day-to-day behaviour it may be because the daily routine of existence makes little call on his best powers. We recognise too that temperamental qualities also are not unaffected, that the reduction in self-criticism may lead to tactless and inconsiderate behaviour, and that the more immediate translation of thought and feeling into action can show itself in errors of judgement. The damage, once done, is irreparable. . . .
>
> Sargant and Slater (1944)

Both insulin therapy and lobotomies were slowly phased out as treatments for the mentally ill, but another of the physical therapies introduced in the mid twentieth century, electric shock (ECT) remains in use to this day largely because it has been found to be effective in a number of studies (see next chapter). This treatment, introduced by Cerletti and Bini in the late 1930s, consists of producing convulsions in a patient by means of passing an electric current through two electrodes placed on the forehead. The idea that such convulsions might help the mentally ill patient was not new; as long ago as 1798, for example, Weickhardt had recommended the giving of camphor to the point of producing vertigo and epileptic fits.

ECT was (and is) used primarily in the treatment of patients with severe depression. Early claims for its effectiveness bordered on the miraculous. Batt (1943), for example, reported a recovery rate of 87%. Fitzgerald (1943) was only slightly less optimistic, suggesting the figure was 78%. In neither report, however was there any attempt to gather data on recovery rates in concurrent controls. Despite this, other psychiatrists accepted the quoted recovery rates as an indication of the effectiveness of ECT. Typical is the following quotation from Napier (1944):

> It is a remarkable advance that a type of case in which the outlook was formerly so problematical can now be offered with some confidence the prospect of restoration in a matter of weeks

Some researchers attempted to evaluate ECT by comparing their results with those from *historical controls* (see Chapter 2) or from concurrent patients who for one reason or another had not been offered the treatment of choice (ECT). But such studies largely only illustrated the weaknesses of such an approach. That by Karagulla (1950), for example, compared results for six groups of patients. Two groups, men and women, had been treated at the Royal Edinburgh Hospital for Mental and Nervous Disorders in the years 1900–39 (before the advent of ECT). The other four groups had been treated in the years 1940–48, two (men and women) by ECT and two others (men and women) not using ECT. It requires little imagination to suppose that the historical controls seen during the period 1900–39 are of little use in evaluating ECT; any difference between the recovery rates for the periods 1900–39 and 1940–48 in favour of the latter, could be explained by many other factors than treatment with ECT. The differences between the ECT groups and the concurrent controls are also virtually impossible to assess since the decision to use ECT on a patient was a subjective one by the clinicians involved. There is no way of knowing whether the treated and untreated groups are comparable. (More comments and criticisms of historical control studies will be found in the next chapter.)

A scientifically acceptable study of the benefits or otherwise of ECT had to wait until 1965 as we shall recount in Chapter 2. At the end of the 1940s and the beginning of the 1950s, the physical treatments introduced into psychiatry 30 years earlier still formed the core of most psychiatrists treatment armoury. But matters were about to change; in the 1950s several entirely new types of drugs were to be introduced in psychiatric practice. In the main the discovery of these drugs was not based on a scientific knowledge of brain chemicals, rather their discovery was for the most part serendipity, resulting from acute observations made by clinicians such as Henri Laborit (the effects of the antihistamine promethazine, from which developed chlorpromazine), and John Cade who first described the value of lithium in manic depression by observing its effect on a number of patients. The tricyclic antidepressants and the Selective Serotonin Reuptake Inhibitors or SSRIs which had fewer side-effects in treating depression were also discovered in the 1950s. Finally, almost by accident, Leo Sternback in 1957 identified the benzodiazepines for treating mild anxiety.

The need to establish whether or not these newly discovered compounds were effective in treating mentally disturbed patients, greatly increased most psychiatrist's appreciation of the need for acceptable procedures for evaluating treatments. And after 1960 the increasing need to satisfy regulatory authorities (prior to 1960 only the USA had such a body, overseeing the introduction of new drugs into general use, but the thalidomide tragedy changed the situation dramatically) meant that the controlled clinical trial, the subject of Chapter 2, increasingly became viewed as the 'gold standard' for evaluating competing therapies. A quotation from one of the psychiatric champions of this approach, Michael Shepherd (1959), remains almost the perfect model for the modern scientific view that psychiatrists should have in the evaluation of psychotropic drug therapies, in particular, and in the evaluation of psychiatric treatments in general:

> The clinician is compelled to hold the balance between the scales of laboratory data on the one hand and stochastic theory on the other. Though his experience and judgement are essential it will be necessary for him to adopt a more experimental role in the future if he is to co-operate fully with the pharmacologist and the statistician whose techniques he should understand if full weight is to be given to observations made in the clinical setting.

1.3 Summary

In the last 50–60 years medicine has made giant strides in finding effective treatments for a range of conditions. In the 1940s, for example, death in childhood from polio, diphtheria, and whooping cough were commonplace but is now thankfully rare (at least in most of Europe and the USA). And the treatment of the mentally ill has also made great progress. Drug treatment of schizophrenia, depression, and anxiety disorders have been found to be effective and have done much to alleviate the misery of these conditions. Drug treatment of mental illness works by altering in some way the chemistry of the body. Chlorpromazine, for example, has been shown to interfere with the action of the neurotransmitter dopamine. But the modern view of mental illness, that it has both psychological and physical dimensions, implies that effective treatment must aim to ease the suffering of the mind as well as correcting possible abnormalities of chemistry. And so, in the 1970s, behavioural psychotherapy began to be used to treat particular disorders. More recently cognitive therapy has been introduced. This provides a simple, straightforward treatment regimen which lasts weeks rather than years, and above all permits the patients to make sense of, and thus hopefully control, their psychological problems.

A cornerstone of the improvements in treatment in medicine in general and psychiatry in particular has been the introduction of an acceptable scientific approach to treatment evaluation, i.e. the clinical trial. Such trials are also the cornerstone of the modern *evidence based medicine* movement (see Sackett *et al.*, 1996). Initially clinical trials in psychiatry largely involved the evaluation of drug treatments as we shall see in Chapter 2. More recently, however, psychological therapies have also been subjected to the rigours of the clinical trial, although there has been a growing awareness that the logistical problems of such trials differ from those of the average drug trial. The reasons why the clinical trial approach is so essential in the evaluation of competing therapies is taken up in Chapter 2.

Chapter 2

The randomized clinical trial

2.1 Introduction

This book is concerned with a fundamental question for psychiatry—how do we tell if a treatment works, is ineffective, or even harmful? If a doctor claims that a certain type of psychotherapy will cure patients of their depression, or a drug company maintains that a new product relieves the symptoms of schizophrenia, how should these assertions be assessed? What sort of evidence do we need to decide that the claims made for the efficacy of clinical treatments are, indeed, valid? One thing is certain: We should not rely on the views of 'experts' unless they produce sound empirical evidence to support their views, nor should we credit the anecdotal evidence of people who have undergone the treatment and, in some cases, have been 'miraculously' cured. One of the principal changes in medical practice and culture during the last one hundred years has been the increasing realization that it is not enough for a doctor to say that his or her treatment works, and nor it is enough for a patient to say likewise. These forms of anecdotal evidence, even if expanded into a series of anecdotes (dignified by the title of case series) are inadequate for the task.

There are many reasons why this is so across medicine, but especially so in psychiatry. Clearly, if one takes a disease like bacterial meningitis, which was 100% fatal, and then introduce penicillin, after which it becomes almost 100% curable, assuming treatment is given in a timely fashion, a series of case reports is sufficient to establish benefit, and no one would even dream of experimenting further. Likewise, the treatment of cardiac arrest would come under the same heading. However, this situation has never yet applied to psychiatry, and we suspect never will. Why not?

First of all, many disorders in psychiatry improve spontaneously. Thus any treatment that the patient may have received is likely to be credited for this improvement by both patient and doctor. This accounts for much of the success of alternative therapies throughout history. Lest we forget, generations and generations of physicians would, in all honesty, have reported that bleeding was an effective treatment, and would be supported in this claim by those patients lucky enough to survive the intervention. Thus in any disorder which is not universally fatal, anecdotal opinion alone will invariably support any treatment claim.

Second, this process of spontaneous recovery is accentuated by what is called 'regression to the mean'. Let us take a disorder in which symptoms wax and wane, such as depression, asthma, or arthritis. People tend to go to see the doctor when their symptoms are worse. Inevitably symptoms improve over time, as this is the natural history of the condition. However, the physician will falsely conclude that his or her intervention was responsible for this improvement, unaware of the fact that he or she is usually seeing the patient at their worst. For this reason regression to the mean is also called 'the physician's friend'.

Third are the 'non specific' effects of treatment, which may also include the *placebo effect*. The simple act of taking an interest in some one, listening to them, paying attention and giving them the expectation that you will do something, anything, is itself a powerful intervention. For that reason many charismatic doctors have, over the years, claimed great success for their particular treatment, whatever it may be, when the 'real' intervention is essentially their own personality. A powerful example of the placebo effect in action is provided by the work of the French psychiatrist Heinz Lehmann who studied three of the most deteriorated schizophrenics in an old asylum in Verdun. Nursing staff and patients were told that the patients were going to be given a new experimental hormone by injection. The injection site was painted with a disinfectant that left a prominent red stain. After three weeks, two of the three patients had begun to talk and were talking rationally. The injection was a placebo. (Lehmann, 1993)

Fourth is selection bias. If one offers a treatment to a hundred people, not all of them accept. Often in psychiatry only a small proportion actually do. But this proportion is not random, and will almost invariably contain an over representation of those with a good prognosis anyway. It may include those with more stable backgrounds, less severe illness, less comorbidity (such as drugs or alcohol), a greater chance of a job to return to, a more supportive home environment, and so on and so forth. Any or all of these might be associated with both the decision to accept treatment, and a better prognosis anyway. Thus if someone gets better on Treatment A it may be that Treatment A actually works, or it may be that those who accepted Treatment A were those more likely to improve irrespective of treatment. All of these factors that are associated both with the decision to accept treatment, and the outcome of the treatment as well, are alternative explanations for why the treatment seems to work. The technical term for such factors is *confounders*.

Take the question of whether or not the introduction of the Samaritans has reduced the suicide rate. A study was performed looking at the change in the rate of suicide in a number of British towns that opened a branch of the Samaritans. It is clear that there was indeed a considerable reduction in the suicide rate in those towns, and it happened at around the time that the Samaritan branches were opened. On first sight there is strong evidence for an effect of the Samaritans on suicide rates (Fig. 2.1) But in Fig. 2.2 we see what happened to the suicide rate in those towns that did *not* introduce a Samaritans branch during the same period.

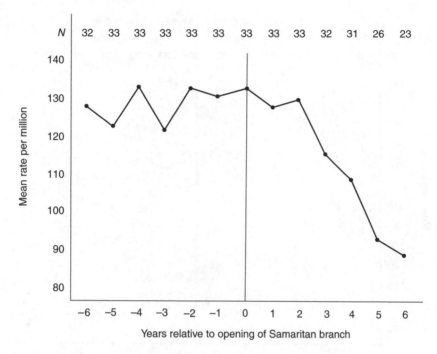

Fig. 2.1 Suicide rates in towns in which Samaritan branches opened.

It is clear that there was a similar decrease in suicide rates in those towns as well. The reason for the general decrease in suicides was almost certainly the switch from domestic to natural gas, which happened at about the same time as the Samaritans became established. Thus the change in gas is a confounder—it is associated both with a fall in the suicide rate, and also with the introduction of the Samaritans, and causes a perceived association between the intervention and the response. Of course, that is not to say that the Samaritans did not do an excellent job—simply that we cannot ascribe the fall in suicide rate at that time to their presence.

So if anecdote and number of people successfully treated alone is no real guide, how can we decide if a specific treatment works or not? We need to *experiment*, a fact recognized over 50 years ago by Pickering in his 1949 Presidential address to the Section of Experimental Medicine and Therapeutics of the Royal Society of Medicine:

> Therapeutics is the branch of medicine that, by its very nature, should be experimental. For if we take a patient affected with a malady, and we alter his conditions of life, either by dieting him, or putting him to bed, or by administering to him a drug, or by performing on him an operation, we are performing an experiment. And if we are scientifically minded we should record the results. Before concluding that the change for better or for worse in the patient is due to the specific treatment employed, we must ascertain whether the result can be repeated a significant number of times in similar patients, whether the result was merely due to the natural history of the disease, or in other words to the lapse of time, or whether it was due

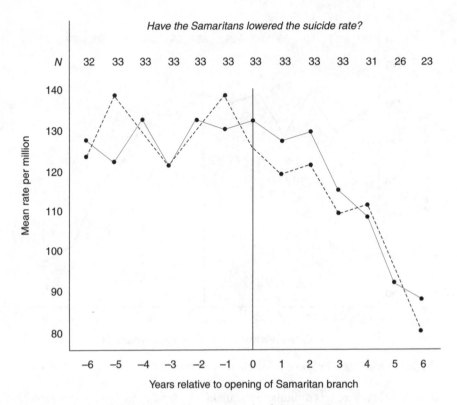

Fig. 2.2 Suicide rates in towns without a branch of the Samaritans.

to some other factor which was necessarily associated with the therapeutic measure in question. And if, as a result of these procedures, we learn that the therapeutic measure employed produces a significant, though not very pronounced improvement, we would experiment with the method, altering dosage or other detail to see if it can be improved. This would seem the procedure to be expected of men with six years of scientific training behind them. But it has not been followed. Had it been done we should have gained a fairly precise knowledge of the place of individual methods of therapy in disease, and our efficiency as doctors would have been enormously enhanced.

Pickering (1949)

The experimental procedure needed in the evaluation of competing treatments is the clinical trial.

2.2 The clinical trial

The clinical trial is a medical experiment designed to evaluate which (if any) of two or more treatments is the more effective. It is based on one of the oldest principles of scientific investigation, namely that new information is obtained from a comparison of alternate states. The three main components of a clinical trial are:

- Comparison of a group of patients given the treatment under investigation (the *treatment group*) with another group of patients given either an older or standard treatment, if one exists, or an 'inert treatment' generally known as a placebo (the *control group*). (Some trials may, of course, involve several treatment groups and a control group, but it eases this general discussion to concentrate on the simple two-group situation.)

- A method of assigning patients to the treatment and control groups.

- A means of assessing effectiveness, i.e. a measure of *outcome*—this may range from a simple rating of 'improved/not improved' to a numerical measure of some characteristic of the patient such as their depression. Most trials in psychiatry will involve several measures of outcome. (Outcome measures for psychiatric trials are considered in Chapter 3.)

2.2.1 The control group

The way to improve a treatment is to eliminate controls

Hugo Muench—quoted in Meinert (1986)

A control group is a necessary component of a clinical trial in order to overcome some of the problems mentioned in the introduction, for example, spontaneous recovery. Members of the control group need to be assessed over the same time period and under similar conditions as the patients in the treatment group to avoid problems of bias etc. The results from a trial in which the enrolment to, and the administration of the test and comparison treatments is *not* concurrent, are likely to be far less convincing, although they may overcome certain ethical problems perceived as important by some clinicians (see later in the chapter). An example is provided by the use of *historical controls*. With this approach all suitable patients receive the new treatment and their outcomes are compared with those extracted from the records of patients previously given the standard treatment (the historical controls). The problems of such a study are well documented (see, for example, Everitt and Pickles, 2000), and include:

- Past observations are unlikely to relate to a precisely similar group of patients as those currently receiving the new treatment.

- The quality of information extracted from the historical control patients is likely to be different (probably inferior) than that collected from the patients being given the new treatment, since they were not initially intended to be part of a treatment comparison.

- Patients given a new, and as yet unproven treatment, are likely to be far more closely monitored, and receive more intensive ancillary care than the historical control patients, who received the orthodox treatment in routine circumstances. Any observed difference in outcome between the two groups might be due to this extra care given to the current patients rather than a real treatment difference.

Such problems generally lead to studies that use historical controls for assessing the effectiveness of competing treatments, exaggerating the effectiveness of the new treatment—see, for example, Sacks *et al.* (1983). (Early naturalistic studies in which ill people were given a treatment, and the treatment declared effective if many became well, use *implicit* historical controls, namely those people who went untreated.)

2.2.2 Treatment assignment in clinical trials

One of the most important aspects of a clinical trial is the question of how patients should be allocated to the treatment group and control group. As Silverman (1985) states:

> How is the impossible decision made to choose between the accepted standard treatment and the proposed improved approach when a fellow human being must be assigned to one of the two (or more) treatments under test? Despite the most extensive pre-clinical studies, the first human allocation of a powerful treatment is largely a blind gamble and it is perhaps not surprising that so much has been written on the most appropriate fashion to allocate treatments in a trial.

The objective in allocation is that the treatment group and control group should be alike in all respects except the treatment received. As a result, the clinical trial is more likely to provide an unbiased comparison of the difference between the two treatments. Let's begin by considering some flawed allocation procedures that are unlikely to achieve the desired degree of similarity of the two groups:

- Perhaps, the clinician should decide which patient goes into which group? Possibly, but then the results of the trial would be viewed with a considerable amount of scepticism. The clinician, might, for example, allocate the patients with the worst prognosis to the, in his or her opinion, 'promising' new therapy and the better ones to the older treatment, no doubt with the best possible intention in respect of her patients. Or older patients might receive the traditional therapy and youngsters the new one, and so on. All of these procedures would tend to invalidate the results from the trial.

- Should the patients themselves decide what treatment to receive? Again this would be highly undesirable. They are likely to believe that the new therapy is about to solve all of their problems. Why else would it be featuring in the trial? What patient would knowingly select a placebo?

- So perhaps, the first patients to volunteer to take part in the trial should all be given the novel treatment, for example, and the later ones used as controls? Again early volunteers might be more seriously ill, those desperate to find a new remedy that works.

- So what about putting alternative patients into each group? The objection to this is that the clinician will know who is receiving what treatment and may be tempted to 'tinker' with the scheme to ensure that his patients who are most ill receive the new treatment.

So how should we form treatment and control groups? The answer is deceptively simple—use *randomization*. The group to which a participant in the trial is allocated is decided by chance. It *could* be arranged by flipping a coin each time a new eligible patient arrives, and allocating the patient to the new treatment if the result is a head, or to the control group if a tail appears. In practice of course, a more sophisticated randomization procedure will be used, as we shall see in the next chapter. The essential feature for now, however, is the randomization rather than the mechanism used to achieve it.

Whereas the use of comparison groups for detecting differential health effects has a long history, going back over 2000 years to the book of Daniel (see Ederer, 1998) randomization was introduced into scientific experiments far more recently, when in 1926 RA (later Sir Ronald) Fisher randomly assigned individual blocks or plots of land in agricultural experiments to receive particular types of 'treatment'—different amounts of fertilizer. (In fact Fisher may have been nearly three hundred years behind the times when he advocated randomization since according to Chalmers, 2001, the first exposition of random allocation came from the Flemish physician Jean Baptiste van Helmont, writing in 1662, in which he advocated casting lots to decide which patients should receive blood-letting and which would not, and that the outcome measure would be the number of funerals in each group. However, there is no evidence that any contemporary physician accepted the challenge!)

The experimental studies in medicine carried out prior to Fisher's introduction of randomization generally employed alternate allocation in which as we now know the clinician has ample opportunity to guess and hence possibly alter treatment allocation. Examples include:

- In 1816, army surgeon Alexander Hamilton apparently used alternate allocation in a further attempt to ascertain the effectiveness or otherwise use of blood-letting, although later historians have cast doubts on whether or not he ever did the experiments as reported.

- The work of Thomas Balfour at the Royal Military Asylum in Chelsea in 1854. Balfour was unimpressed by the claims made of the ability of a homeopathic medicine to prevent scarlet fever in the orphan boys in his care. He gives the following account of how he set about investigating the claim:

There were 151 boys of whom I had tolerably satisfactory evidence that they had not had scarlatina: I divided them into two sections, taking them alternately from the list, to prevent the imputation of selection. To the first section (76) I gave belladonna: to the second (75) I gave none: the result was that two in each section were attacked by the disease. The numbers are too small to justify deductions as to the prophylactic power of belladonna, but the observation is good, because it shows how apt we are to be misled by imperfect observation. Had I given the remedy to all of the boys, I should probably have attributed to it the cessation of the epidemic

Apart from the flawed allocation procedure, everything else for a sound experiment is there; the need for sound eligibility criteria (boys who had not yet had scarlet fever), the problem of Type 2 errors (Balfour considered that his numbers were too small, and there remained a chance that Belladonna did prevent scarlet fever, albeit very weakly), and the very real and tangible risk of drawing an incorrect inference from uncontrolled data (the epidemic would appear to have been either over, or less virulent than previously thought, leading physicians to falsely believe that the relative absence of scarlet fever in the orphanage was due to belladonna).

- The work of William Fletcher, who demonstrated the role of polished rice in the aetiology of beri beri, and how this could be overcome by using uncured rice. He did so by alternative allocation of patients who were inmates of the 'lunatic asylum' in Kuala Lumpur.
- The evaluation of serum treatment for lobar pneumonia in 1934 (Chalmers *et al.*, 2002), and the treatment trial of the common cold carried out during wartime by Philip D'Arcy Hart (the 'patulin' trial, MRC, 1944) employed alternate allocation.

The modern clinical trial, as we know it, began immediately after the Second World War, when Austin Bradford Hill began the now routine practice of allocation concealment with true randomized, rather than alternate, allocation. Contrary to the popular perception the first such trial was not the Medical Research Council trial of streptomycin for pulmonary tuberculosis, but another MRC trial of the new whooping cough vaccine. However, that trial did not report until 1951, whilst the more famous streptomycin trial reported in 1948 (MRC, 1948), and thus has received all the plaudits (Doll, 1998).

It is interesting to read Sir Richard Doll's recollections of that epochal trial (Doll, 1998). The MRC Committee faced several ethical dilemmas. First, given that streptomycin was potentially a lifesaver, certainly if one believed the animal experiments, could they withhold treatment at all? The answer was yes, since supplies were very limited indeed, and there was no possibility that everyone who might benefit from treatment could receive the drug anyway (there was a thriving black market for the drug, which was widely available only in the USA). In fact that raised a second moral issue—should they use all their supplies on the treatment of military tuberculosis and tuberculosis meningitis, which were invariably fatal? They did not, but did begin non-randomized uncontrolled trials in both conditions at the same time (reminding us that it is unethical and unnecessary to randomize to an inactive treatment in a condition that is invariably fatal, a situation which fortunately does not concern us in psychiatry—*vide infra*). Second, they decided that informed consent was not necessary from the participants. Bradford Hill argued against it, pointing that informed consent was rarely obtained in routine clinical practice anyway. In echoes of an argument to which we will return, he said that as clinicians did not seek informed consent before giving a new treatment non randomly to their patients, it seemed unfair to impose this requirement when the clinician was now attempting to test the drug in a way which would benefit generations of patients to come. Bradford Hill was raising the question of double standards, a question that remains valid today. Instead, as Sir Richard Doll recollects, the 'over riding issue [for the committee] was the welfare of the patient'. Times were of course different in the post war years, when the notion of self-sacrifice for the common good was stronger than now. It is however untrue to say, as some have, that informed consent simply did not exist during that period. The MRC did use written informed consent in the whooping cough trial that preceded the streptomycin trial—supplies of the vaccine were not limited, and many children would be exposed to the vaccine *during* the trial who would not actually develop whooping cough, even if one could not predict who they were.

The first psychiatrist to advocate the use of Fisher's experimental approach for the evaluation of psychiatric treatments, particularly the physical treatments described in Chapter 1, appears to have been Sir Aubrey Lewis (1946). In his paper he criticizes past studies and of a controlled clinical trial he concludes:

> An organised experiment would demand much that hitherto has not been practicable, including voluntary acceptance by independent hospitals and clinics of an agreed procedure for the selection, management, evaluation of mental state, and follow-up investigation of treated, as well as of control cases. Such an experiment, as R.A. Fisher has demonstrated, requires much forethought and self-discipline on the part of those who carry it out.

It is unclear who carried out the first truly randomized controlled trial in psychiatry. Healy (1997) gives us four candidates:

- A placebo controlled randomly allocated trial of chlorpromazine for treating schizophrenia carried out in 1954 in Birmingham, UK, by the husband and wife team of Joel and Charmain Elkes (Elkes, 1954).

- Again in 1954, a trial performed by Linford Rees who randomly allocated 100 anxious patients to either placebo of chlorpromazine (Rees, 1956).

- A trial undertaken at the Maudsley Hospital in London by David Davies and Michael Shepherd to study the use of reserpine for treating depression. This trial began in 1953 but reports of it did not appear until Davies and Shepherd (1955). (Ironically, most modern psychiatrists who have heard of reserpine will associate it with producing, rather than alleviating depression!)

- Finally during the same time period Morgens Schou and Eric Stromgren used a randomized trial and showed the effectiveness of lithium as a treatment for mania. (Schou et al., 1954)

Since trials take place over many months and indeed, in some cases, years, perhaps it is invidious to try to label any one trial as the first in psychiatry. But certainly by the 1960s, trials in psychiatry had become far more ambitious and complex than those undertaken a few years earlier. The UK Medical Research Council clinical trial of the treatment of depressive illness illustrates the change. This trial, the results of which were published in 1965, was hailed as a landmark study and as a 'breakthrough in psychiatry's aspirations to free itself from complete reliance on empiricism'. The trial, which was conducted in three geographically dispersed regions within the UK, involved some 55 psychiatrists, recruited 269 patients with depression, randomized them to one of four treatment groups (two classes of antidepressant drug, ECT, and a placebo), and then followed them for almost six months. The personnel associated with the trial now reads like a Who's Who of British psychiatry and statistics and included, Robert Cawley, Archie Cochrane and Austin Bradford Hill.

We can now return to consideration of why randomization is the allocation method of choice. There are a variety of reasons:

- It provides an impartial method of allocating patients to treatments free from possible personal biases. In other words randomization deals with the selection bias problem identified in the introduction of this chapter. It ensures that like is being compared with like, and that hidden biases favouring one arm of the trial or the other have not crept in.

♦ Randomization deals directly with confounders by ensuring that they are distributed randomly (and hence without bias) between those who do, and those who do not, receive the treatment. And here lies the real beauty of randomization; it deals with not only the confounders that you *had* thought of and possibly even recorded, but also with those that you *had not!* (Sibbald and Roland, 1998). For example, you might be aware that response to a particular intervention is better in females than males. Gender would then be a confounder, since if you had one arm of the trial that had more females than males, then that treatment would falsely appear to be superior. You *could* deal with the situation by requiring that the two arms have equal numbers of males and females, and thus eliminate the effect of the confounder, although if the trial was large enough you could reasonably rely on randomization alone to take care of the problem. But much is mysterious in psychiatry, and we can say with confidence that there is much we do not know about why some people respond better to any given treatment than others. Here is the elegance of randomization—it will take care of these 'mystery' confounders so that you no longer need to worry about them, either now, or in the future, not least when you submit your papers!

♦ Randomization provides a firm basis for the application of the statistical methodology likely to be needed when evaluating the results from a trial. Technically it provides a probabilistic basis for inference from the observed results when considered in reference to all possible results.

And what happens if you don't randomize? The answer is simple. You are more likely to come up with the wrong answer. In a series of studies, it has been established beyond all doubt that when you don't randomize, all sorts of biases creep in (Antman *et al.*, 1992; Chalmers *et al.*, 1977; Chalmers *et al.*, 1983; Kleijnen *et al.*, 1997; Sacks *et al.*, 1982; Sacks *et al.*, 1987; Schultz *et al.*, 1994; Schultz *et al.*, 1995). And what these biases do is to systematically over state the effectiveness of the new treatment. Study after study that compares the results of evaluations of new treatments that do not include randomization, find that these designs are far more likely to report that the new treatment works. Now it could be that for some perverse reason doctors tend to perform randomized controlled trials on weaker, less effective treatments, reserving the inferior research designs for the more powerful treatments. However, one can show the same even within randomized controlled trials—the better the design of the trial, and the greater the protection from bias, the less the chance of showing that the new treatment works. We will return to this theme later in this chapter when we consider allocation concealment, and again in our concluding chapter, Chapter 8.

An example of how randomization overcomes unrealistic optimism comes from the literature on psychological 'debriefing' (Raphael *et al.*, 1995). Debriefing is a procedure that was introduced over the last two decades as a simple procedure to be used in the aftermath of trauma, with the aim of educating people about likely reactions and symptoms. The purpose of debriefing is to reduce current distress and to prevent the onset of post traumatic stress disorder (PTSD). It is an intervention that is intuitively appealing, particularly in circumstances where people feel the need to 'do something'. But how do we know if it works? If we simply asked the people carrying out the debriefing, there is not a shadow of doubt they would, and do, say that it is an excellent intervention, and they feel they are doing good. Indeed, such is the popularity of the intervention that in some organizations it has become compulsory where staff members are exposed to trauma. If we asked those who took part, then again the studies show that most are very satisfied with debriefing, and felt the experience was beneficial. Of course, some do go on to develop psychiatric disorders despite debriefing, but supporters of debriefing would say that the intervention is not perfect, and that these people were going to get PTSD anyway.

It is only when researchers starting doing randomized controlled trials that a different picture emerged. One of us (SW) was involved in a systematic review of the literature for the Cochrane Collaboration (Wessely et al., 2000). The results were not what the advocates (and there were many) of debriefing expected. When one compared those who received single session debriefing to those who by chance alone (randomization) did not, there was no evidence at all that debriefing reduced psychological distress or prevented PTSD (Litz et al., 2002; Wessely et al., 2000). Worse, the two trials with the longest follow up both reported something unexpected—that the rate of PTSD was significantly higher in those who had been debriefed. Armed with that information we can now start to make suggestions as to why debriefing not only didn't work, but actually made some people worse. But the important point to note is that it is not enough that an intervention 'feels good', nor that participants think it is good. It is only from randomized controlled trials that we can see the real picture, and without those trials in this case we would never have learnt that this apparently 'good thing', debriefing, might do harm.

Random allocation by ensuring a lack of selection bias, and distributing both known and unknown confounders impartially amongst the treatment and control groups, goes a long way to making the interpretation of an observed difference unambiguous—its cause is very likely to be the different treatments received by the patients in the two groups; a long way, but not the whole way.

2.2.3 Allocation concealment and Blinding

Unfortunately, saying that a trial is 'randomized' is not in itself a complete protection against all forms of potential bias. Randomization must be combined with *allocation concealment* and, if possible, *blinding*. Allocation concealment and blinding are often confused, but are different. The former refers to methods of preventing any interference with the assignment of treatment during the randomization process, the latter to who has knowledge of what treatment is being given or received as the trial progresses. Allocation concealment is therefore a defence against selection bias, whilst blinding reduces observer and other information biases. The two also have different histories—blindness has been recognized as an important part of valid treatment assessments for over two hundred years (Kaptchuk, 1998), whilst allocation concealment is just over 50 years old (Chalmers, 2001).

The randomized controlled trial is now generally regarded as the 'gold standard' in the world of clinical trials, but not all randomized trials are equal. Assessing the quality of allocation concealment has become a key aspect of assessing the quality of a trial. The reason is because there is a considerable literature that suggests that given the chance, clinicians can and do deliberately try to overcome the constraints on choosing treatments for particular patients imposed by the randomized design. This mostly arises when the clinician has a view as to which of the two treatments is preferable, or already believes that the treatment is effective, and is unhappy about the possibility of a patient receiving a placebo. In the other direction, clinicians have been known to feel that a particular patient whilst fulfilling the criteria for the trial is still too unwell for the new treatment, and acts to ensure they receive the old (Schultz and Grimes, 2002). It is not unknown for envelopes containing randomization codes to be held up to the light and then the sequence altered to ensure the 'right' treatment is allocated. Even alleged opaque envelopes have been X-rayed in an effort to reveal their contents (Schultz and Grimes, 2002)! Ringing a telephone randomization service, which should be fool proof, can be subverted if the clinician asks for, and receives, several randomization codes at once. Clinicians indulging in such behaviour might consider their reasons 'honourable', but the result is likely to be very damaging to the validity of the trial, undermining not only the efforts of all the others involved in running the trial, but also probably wasting the time of the patients themselves. That this is so is clear from the evidence that trials in which concealment of treatment is either inadequate or unclear, alter the treatment effect in unpredictable ways (Kunz and Oxman, 1998), although, in general the problem leads to a systematic bias in favour of the new treatment (Schulz *et al.*, 1994, 1995). It is for this reason that we place considerable importance on adequate allocation concealment. Practical steps to achieve this are described in Appendix A.

Blinding is distinct from allocation concealment. The latter ensures the purity of the treatment assignment, and is necessary for all well conducted trials including those in mental health. Blinding concerns the degree in which patients, investigators and assessors are kept unaware of what treatment is being received throughout the conduct of the trial. The fundamental idea of blinding in a clinical trial is that the study patients, the people involved with their management, and those collecting the clinical data should not know which treatment a patient is receiving. In this way none of the people mentioned can be influenced by knowledge of the assigned treatment. In practice, different degrees of blinding are often used (or possible)—most common are:

♦ *Single-blind*: the patient only is unaware of which treatment he or she is receiving.

♦ *Double-blind*: both the patient and the investigators (including the treating clinician) are not allowed to know the treatment the patient is receiving.

♦ *Triple blind*: Neither the patient, investigator nor the person(s) responsible for the assessments know the treatment the patient is receiving.

Reasonable allocation concealment is obligatory and should be achieved in all mental health trials. On the other hand, blinding, although desirable, is not always possible; the blinding of physical treatments such as surgery, for example, is often difficult. In such cases a partial solution, at least, is to use a blinded evaluator for recording patients' responses to treatments. Such procedures are particularly applicable when the assessment has a subjective element and when the investigator is likely to recall the treatment given to the patient. For example, in several trials of different psychological therapies for chronic fatigue syndrome (CFS) an assessor blinded to the treatment condition was used, and asked patients not to reveal which treatment they had received to the same assessor (Deale *et al.*, 1997). And Guthrie *et al.* (1993) describe a randomized controlled trial of psychotherapy against supportive listening in patients with irritable bowel syndrome, in which both the psychiatrists and the patients knew which group they were in. But the outcomes (psychological and bowel symptoms) were assessed by another psychiatrist and a gastroenterologist who were blind to treatment allocation.

Finally, it has to be admitted that in truth, blinded treatment administration, however carefully arranged, is rarely 100% effective. All forms of treatment, but particularly drugs, can produce side-effects and tell-tale signs that may serve to identify the treatment being used to the clinicians and other researchers involved with the trial. Trial designers need to be realistic about this possibility, trying hard to eliminate it, but being on the look out that it has occurred. The problem is considered in more detail in Basoğlu *et al.* (1997).

2.2.4   Types of clinical trial

Not all clinical trials are the same. There are, for example, *therapeutic trials*, in which a new therapy, such as a pharmaceutical agent (drug) is compared to a conventional therapy, and *placebo-controlled* clinical trials where a group of patients treated with a new treatment are compared to a group who receive a placebo control. In some cases the intervention being assessed is an entire system of care that might include several different interventions. This is particularly common in psychiatry and an example is the UK-700 trial of case management for schizophrenia (UK 700 Group: Creed F, 1999). Such trials are often referred to as *pragmatic* (see Schwartz and Lellouch, 1967), since the innovation consists of two or more possible agents or procedures used in combination, so that it is not possible to identify the mechanism by which the new procedure produces its effects. But the argument generally made for such a study is that conclusive evidence that the new combined therapeutic approach is indeed beneficial in practice is adequate for its adoption even when the mechanism of the effect is unknown.

A pragmatic trial focuses on the question 'what is the better treatment in the particular clinical circumstances of the patients in the study?' and aim to measure effectiveness, the benefit a treatment produces in routine clinical practice. In contrast, what is known as an *explanatory trial* attempts to measure treatment efficacy, the benefit a treatment produces under ideal conditions. We shall return to the implications of this pragmatic/explanatory division for psychiatric trials, in later chapters.

The pharmaceutical industry uses a well-established taxonomy of clinical trials involving drug therapy, in which the categories are as follows (after Pocock, 1983):

Phase I trials: clinical pharmacology and toxicity

These first experiments in man are primarily concerned with drug safety, not efficacy, and hence are usually performed on healthy, human volunteers, often pharmaceutical company employees. The first objective is to determine an acceptable single drug dosage (i.e. how much drug can be given without causing serious side-effects). Such information is often obtained from *dose-escalation* experiments, whereby a volunteer is subjected to increasing doses of the drug according to a predetermined schedule. Phase I will also include studies of drug metabolism and bioavailability and later, studies of multiple doses will be undertaken to determine appropriate dose schedules for use in phase II. (These are often called 'first into man' trials.) After studies in normal volunteers, the initial trials in patients will also be of phase I type. Typically, phase I studies might require a total of around 20–80 subjects or patients. The general aim of such studies is to provide a relatively clear picture of a drug, but one that will require refinement during phases II and III. In brief, phase I trials are concerned with safety and dosing.

Phase II trials: initial clinical investigation for treatment effect

These (usually non-randomized) trials are conducted to provide a preliminary indication of the potential activity of a new drug or other type of therapy. They are generally fairly small-scale investigations that involve close monitoring of each patient. Phase II trials can sometimes be set up as a screening process to select out those relatively few drugs of genuine potential from the larger number of drugs which are inactive or over-toxic, so that the chosen drugs may proceed to phase III trials. Seldom will phase III go beyond 100–200 patients on a drug. The primary goals of phase II trials are:

◆ to identify accurately the patient population that can benefit from the drug,

◆ to verify and estimate the effectiveness of the dosing regimen determined in Phase I.

Phase III trials: full-scale evaluation of treatment

After a drug is shown to be reasonably effective, it is essential to compare it with the current standard treatment(s) for the same condition in a large trial involving a substantial number of patients and which uses random allocation. To some people the term 'clinical trial' is synonymous with such a full-scale phase III trial, which is the most rigorous and extensive type of scientific clinical investigation of a new treatment. It is in a phase III trial that the efficacy and/or effectiveness of a treatment is assessed.

Phase IV trials: postmarketing surveillance

After the research programme leading to a drug being approved for marketing, there remain substantial enquiries still to be undertaken as regards monitoring for adverse effects and additional large-scale, long-term studies of morbidity and mortality.

This book will be largely concerned with phase III trials. In order to accumulate enough patients in a time short enough to make a trial viable, many clinical trials will involve recruiting patients at more than a single centre (for example, different clinics, different hospitals, etc.) and are known as *multicentre trials*. The principal advantage of carrying out a multicentre trial is that patient accrual is much quicker so that the trial can be made larger and the planned number of patients can be achieved more quickly. The end-result should be that a multi-centre trial reaches more reliable conclusions at a faster rate, so that overall progress in the treatment of a given disease is enhanced. We consider multicentre trials further in Chapter 3. (As well as the different types of trial described above, there are also different *designs* that may be used for clinical trials, a point we shall also discuss in Chapter 3.)

2.3 Ethical issues in clinical trials

Randomization is a marvellously elegant solution to the problem of allocating patients to treatments in a clinical trial. But the elegance of the procedure cannot disguise that it poses possible ethical dilemmas for clinicians and also often raises concern amongst individuals who are prospective participants in a trial. Some clinicians have argued that allowing chance to be the determining factor when assigning treatment to patients has no place in medicine, and that only a physician can decide which treatment a patient should receive, using his or her best judgement. Perhaps they find it difficult to swallow that the objectivity of randomization is more likely to get at the truth than the subjective impressions generated from clinical experience. (After all, the implication of accepting that this is so is that the clinician must necessarily defer to the authority of the statistician!) And the patient being recruited for a trial, having been made aware of the randomization component, might reasonably be troubled by the possibility of receiving an 'inferior' treatment.

Clearly if the clinician is aware that one treatment is superior to another, or to no treatment, then randomization is unethical. The Declaration of Helsinki makes it clear that the physician must act in the patient's interest, and cannot withhold an effective treatment, nor give a treatment that he knows will worsen the patient's condition. No trial has ever been performed to prove that penicillin is effective for meningitis and no doctor would have considered taking part if any such trial had ever been suggested. But such situations are few and far between, and almost entirely absent from psychiatry. The illnesses with which psychiatrists are concerned are usually chronic and wax and wane. Likewise, the treatments with which psychiatrists deal do not have the almost magical properties first seen with the use of penicillin.

When a clinician cannot, in all honesty, say what is the best treatment for his or her patient he or she is then said to be in state of *equipoise*. Most ethicists would agree, in principle, with the concept that it is ethical to employ randomization in a state of true equipoise, provided the patient consents to be a study participant and is fully informed about the potential benefits and risks of the treatments to be compared in the study. The problem is, of course, that many doctors are reluctant to accept the uncertainty about much of what they practice, and are only rarely balanced on the cusp of indifference that is equipoise. Perhaps such doctors need to be reminded of the many, many examples of treatments that so obviously 'worked' that it was a brave person who would ever doubt their efficacy, but are now known to be either useless, or indeed harmful. One of us recalls being a medical SHO and treating cardiac arrthymias with lignocaine. This did indeed stop the appearance of ventricular ectopics, which were thought to be the precursor to ventricular fibrillation, a fatal condition unless immediately reversed. However, randomized trials demonstrated what cardiologists thought impossible—lignocaine killed more patients than it cured.

The history of psychiatry is also littered with claims made for treatments that at one time seemed clearly beneficial, but later proved to be a false dawn. The contemporary debate on debriefing mentioned in Sub-Section 2.2.2 provides a salutary example. One of us (SW) proposed a trial of debriefing some years ago for victims of disaster, but was told in no uncertain terms that this was unethical, since it was so clearly of benefit.

Ethical problems in clinical trials reflect the delicate balance between *individual ethics* and *collective ethics* faced by clinicians. How do they ensure that each individual patient receives the treatment most beneficial for his or her condition, whilst evaluating competing therapies as efficiently as possible so that all future patients might benefit from the superior treatment and, as a consequence, advance public health through careful scientific experimentation? The prime motivation for conducting a trial involves collective ethics, but individual ethics have to be given as much attention as possible without destroying the trial's validity. Naturally the physician's responsibilities to patients during the course of the trial are clear; if the patient's condition deteriorates, the ethical obligation must always and entirely outweigh any experimental conditions. This obligation implies that whenever a doctor thinks that the interests of his or her patient are at stake, the patient must be treated as seen fit. This is an essential requirement for an ethically conducted trial, no matter what complications it may introduce into the final analysis of the data.

A further ethical problem involves the question of when is it justified to use a placebo? This has become particularly important in drug development, since regulatory bodies require that new agents be tested against placebo. But this is often hard to justify. For example, evidence for the effectiveness of existing antidepressants is very strong indeed, and hence entering a patient into a trial in which they might receive a placebo antidepressant gives increasing cause for concern. Drug companies, on the other hand, are reluctant to test their products against active compounds rather than placebos for commercial and marketing reasons.

Some, including the distinguished epidemiologist Rothman, have argued passionately that once an effective treatment is known, there is no place for a placebo condition, and journals should not contemplate publishing such studies (Rothman and Michels, 1994). Rothman then would clearly ban further trials of antidepressants or antipsychotic agents that use placebos.

In contrast the equally distinguished psychiatrist Quitkin argues that the fluctuating nature of psychiatric disorders, the unlikely possibility that delaying treatment will permanently influence outcome, and the very variable placebo rates observed in many psychiatric disorders, means that such an absolutist position should be modified, particularly if, as should always be the case anyway, the placebo group are receiving similar monitoring and general care (Quitkin, 2000). Defenders of the status quo argue strongly that provided participants in the trial who do not respond are given active treatment at a later date, the worst disadvantage that might befall a trial participant is that they have been deprived active treatment for a defined, usually short, period (see, for example, Miller, 2000; Leber, 2000).

Where does this leave us? We believe that if it is indeed true that an effective treatment does exist and is available for the group of patients likely to be the subject of a new clinical trial, then Rothman is correct and there is no justification for a placebo. We note, however, that in many instances the evidence favouring an existing treatment is not as robust as claimed. Likewise, we are aware of the intense arguments about the use of placebos or control conditions in trials, sometimes around AIDS and HIV, in the developing countries. There it is argued, most often by representatives of the countries themselves, that even if a better treatment exists in more developed societies, such treatments are completely out of reach of sufferers in the developing world, whose only chance of getting any medical care or treatment at all is via a randomized controlled trial even if it involves placebo. However, irrespective of the rights and wrongs of the argument, we are unaware of analogous situations in mental health research, although such circumstances might arise in the future. Finally, whilst Quitkin's argument that no permanent damage can be expected if treatment is delayed might be applicable to the situation facing researchers of a new antidepressant, there is evidence starting to emerge that early intervention delays illness progression in the psychoses, which if (and it is a big if) substantiated, means this issue will need to be revisited.

In general the tide is flowing away from the continuing use of placebos to evaluate new treatments when sound evidence exists for the efficacy of the old treatments. In particular, we wonder what is the use of such trials anyway, except to the drug company keen to add a 'me too' drug to the market. There is every reason to support testing new pharmacological compounds in, for example, the field of depression. But to be worthwhile these must now have some inherent benefit over and above the existing and extensive range of antidepressants already available. This might be better efficacy, or rather more likely, improved side effects or safety, but in any event the comparison will need to be with the standard care, which now routinely involves antidepressant medications of proven efficacy.

Those who question the ethics of randomized trials often forget one of the other arguments that are made against clinical trials (particularly explanatory trials), that of their apparent lack of *generalizability* to usual clinical practice. As we will discuss in a later chapter, some opponents of clinical trials frequently point to their 'non real world' setting, and the fact that the results of clinical trials seem often to be 'too good to be true', with the same treatments rarely performing as well in the non trial setting. (In fact evidence for this view is not as solid as one might think as we shall point out later in the book, but the important point to note for the moment is the general belief that patients seem to do better simply because they are in a clinical trial.) Certainly the routine aspects of care are usually performed far more meticulously during the conduct of a trial. Diagnoses are made more precisely. Routine tests are performed more often, and rarely if ever are they forgotten, or the results lost. Follow up is meticulously organized, and great steps taken to ensure that the patient does indeed attend for review. Interventions are explained more carefully, and there is a general air of optimism associated with testing a new intervention that can be missing from routine clinical practice. Consequently the arguments made by those sceptical of the value of clinical trials because of the perceived difficulty of generalizing the findings can, ironically, be used against those who believe that patients may be disadvantaged by being entered into such studies!

It could be argued that there are many circumstances in which it is unethical *not* to do a randomized clinical trial; this argument is enthusiastically supported by the writers of this book, although we recognize that conducting trials that of sufficiently poor quality that they cannot make a meaningful contribution to medical knowledge, is in itself, unethical. The truth is that many of our cherished interventions, or so called 'best practices' have never been rigorously evaluated. There is a very real risk that many things that we do to our patients, or recommend that they do for themselves, may in the fullness of time be found seriously wanting. The greatest danger to patients comes not from those doctors who are prepared to admit both to themselves and to their patients their uncertainty about the best action to take to deal with particular conditions; such people demand to see the evidence for treatment efficacy produced from a high quality randomized trial. Rather it comes from the 'enthusiasts', those clinicians who are so certain that their treatment is the correct one, that they do not entertain the possibility that they might be mistaken. It is a sad and ironic fact that even with the advent of clinical governance, the National Institute for Clinical Excellence (NICE) in the United Kingdom and the like, it remains the case that a clinician can promote a vast range of therapies to his or her patients, and is rarely called to demonstrate the effectiveness or efficacy of what he or she does. If challenged, the old icon of 'clinical freedom' can be invoked, or past experience. Past experience can be misleading, and the plural of anecdote is not evidence. In general there exist very few checks and balances on the clinician, and there is little that can be done to restrain someone from promoting therapies that seem to be based on minimal or no scientific evidence. This is particularly so amongst advocates of alternative therapies (see Chapter 8) and some doctors in private practice.

As Sir Iain Chalmers has memorably pointed out, if one decides to give all ones patients a particular treatment, there are few if any people around who will counsel caution, or even be in a position to stop you. But woe-betide the clinician who admits uncertainty, and so wishes to undertake a clinical trial (Chalmers and Lindley, 2000). 'If I give all my patients the same treatment, no one is around to stop me, but should I decide to give only half of my patients the very same treatment, the world seems full of people who will tell me why I should not do this'—or, to paraphrase Smithells 'I need permission to give a new drug to half my patients, but not to give it to all of them' (Smithells, 1975).

When doctors are able to admit to uncertainty in many of their practices, then no conflict exists between the roles of the doctor and the scientist. In such circumstances it cannot be less ethical to choose a treatment by random allocation within a controlled trial that to choose by what happens to be readily available, hunch, or what a drug company recommends. The most effective argument in favour of randomized clinical trials is that the alternative, practising in complacent uncertainty, is worse. So perhaps the real ethical question is not why randomized clinical trials are undertaken, but why they are not?

2.4 Informed consent

The Nuremberg Code and all subsequent codes covering the ethical requirements for medical experiments involving human beings, have been explicit on the need for voluntary consent (Levine and Lebacqz, 1979; Levine, 1981). A subject's or patient's documented agreement to participate in a clinical trial as a result of having all risks and benefits openly and clearly explained, is known as the patient's *informed consent*. Few clinicians would argue against the need for the voluntary consent of people being asked to take part in a trial, if they are capable of giving it, but there may be less agreement about how much information about the trial should be given to the prospective participant in obtaining his or her consent. Clearly the randomization component of the trial needs to be made clear but how many clinical trial investigators would like to go as far as Berry (1993) in presenting the following document to each possible subject?

> I would like you to participate in a randomized trial. We will in effect flip a coin and give you therapy A if the coin comes up heads and therapy B if it comes up tails. Neither you or I will know what therapy you receive unless problems develop. [After presenting information about the therapies and their possible side-effects:] No one really knows what therapy is better and that is why we're conducting this trial. However, we have had some experience with both therapies, including experience in the current trial. The available data suggest that you will live an average of five months longer on A than on B. But there is substantial variability in the data, and many people who have received B have lived longer than some patients on A. If I were you I would prefer A. My probability that you live longer on A is 25 per cent.
>
> Your participation in this trial will help us treat other patients with this disease, so I ask you in their name. But if you choose not to participate, you will receive whichever therapy you choose, including A or B.

Meinert (1986) stresses that the consent process, to be valid, must be based on factual information presented in an intelligible fashion and in a setting in which the patient is able to make a free choice, without fear or reprisal or prejudicial treatment. Meinert also lists the following general elements of an informed consent:

- A statement that the study involves research, an explanation of the research and the expected duration of the subject's participation, a description of the procedures to be followed, and identification of any procedures that are experimental.

- A description of any foreseeable risks or discomforts to the subject.
- A description of any benefits to the subject or others that may reasonably be expected from the research.
- A disclosure of appropriate alternative procedures or courses of treatment, if any, that might be advantageous to the subject.
- A statement concerning the extent, if any, to which confidentiality of records identifying the subject will be maintained.
- For research involving more than minimal risk, an explanation as to whether any compensation or medical treatments are available if injury occurs and, if so, what they consist of, or where further information may be obtained.
- An explanation of whom to contact for answers to pertinent questions about the research and research subject's rights, and whom to contact in the event of research-related injury.
- A statement that participation is voluntary, refusal to participate will involve no penalty or loss of benefits to which the subject is otherwise entitled, and the subject may discontinue participation at any time without penalty or loss of benefits to which the subject is otherwise entitled.

Informed consent documents should be simply written with terms such as randomization, placebo, masking, etc. being explained in lay terms. We are well aware however, that there is evidence being collected by the Health Technology Assessment Programme on understanding and explaining the meaning of randomization, that suggests that even with the best of intentions and a great deal of effort, it is very difficult to patients to grasp the essence and purpose of the procedure (Featherstone and Donovan, 2002; Lilford, pers. comm). (Perhaps this should not surprise us, since we have a strong impression that many medical professionals likewise are unclear as to the fundamental purpose of randomization!)

Nevertheless, there can be no excusing the use of jargon or obscure language in obtaining consent. But even the clearest consent form may not be understandable by some patients and obtaining informed consent from psychiatric populations has received substantial attention aiming in particular to assess how much such patients understand the risks and benefits of their participation in a trial. Some studies have shown that psychiatric patients, particularly those with the more debilitating mental illnesses such as schizophrenia, are able to understand and use only a portion of the information provided by consent forms. For example, Irwin *et al.* (1985) studied 47 psychotic patients and found that they were able to read the informed consent information presented, and most then reported that their understanding about antipsychotic medication was good. Objective measures, however, did not confirm the patient's self-reports. It appeared that many patients said they understood *only* to mask their confusion over the information provided. (There is evidence that this phenomenon is not restricted to psychiatric patients—see Robinson and Merav, 1976; Leonard *et al.*, 1972.)

Where there is concern that potential participants in a trial cannot understand the information given in informed consent material, it may be acceptable to approach an appropriate individual who is able to consent on the patient's behalf. In general the surrogate should be chosen by the patient, but where this is not possible, it may be acceptable to obtain assent (not consent) from the patient's spouse, parent, adult child, adult sibling or guardian. In the absence of patient choice, these relatives might be expected to be the person's most likely to understand the patient's beliefs and to make decisions that reflect his or her wishes.

The consent process must be completed before any treatment assignment and no patient should be randomized who expresses reluctance or unwillingness to accept whatever treatment is assigned.

Are there circumstances where randomization can take place without consent? A knee jerk response to this question is to say no, and, as we will see when we consider the issue of post randomization consent (the 'Zelen' design), there are many of this opinion. But it is not so simple. First, there is the issue of double standards. Patients give general consent to many aspects of treatment without giving informed consent to each. Second, it is accepted within the Declaration of Helsinki and elsewhere that non-consented trials are permissible in certain well defined circumstances—for example, in research concerning serious illnesses in unconscious patients. We will consider this issue further in the next chapter.

2.5 Compliance

For clinical trial investigators, particularly those working in psychiatry, it is an inescapable fact of life that the participants in their trials often make life difficult by missing appointments, forgetting to take their prescribed treatment from time to time, or not taking it at all but pretending to do so. Such investigators will, no doubt be able to immediately relate to following quotation from Efron (1998):

> There could be no worse experimental animals on earth than human beings; they complain, they go on vacations, they take things they are not supposed to take, they lead incredibly complicated lives, and, sometimes, they do not take their medicine.

Compliance means following both the intervention regimen and trial procedures (for example, clinic visits, laboratory procedures and filling out forms). A non-complier is a patient who fails to meet the standards of compliance as established by the investigator. A high degree of patient compliance is an important aspect of a well-run trial.[1]

But treatment compliance is rarely an all-or-none phenomena. The level of compliance achieved may range from low to high, depending on both the patient and the staff. Perfect compliance is probably impossible to achieve, particularly in drug trials where the patient may be required to take the assigned medication at

---

[1] We note en passant the move away in certain circles from the word 'compliance', as it is alleged to have certain hierarchical overtones, in which patients passively 'comply' with the doctor's 'orders'. Compliance is gradually being replaced by the preferred term adherence. However, compliance remains the favoured term in clinical trial methodology.

the same time of day over long periods of time. Lack of compliance can take a number of forms; the patient may simply dropout of the trial altogether, perhaps, because of some adverse event, or even because they improve and feel they no longer need to take the prescribed medication. Alternatively patients may continue in the trial but take their medication at the wrong time, take extra doses, omit doses, use outdated medication or take the wrong medication.

Level of compliance will depend on a number of factors, including:

♦ the amount of time and inconvenience involved in making follow-up visits to the clinic,

♦ the amount of data being collected,

♦ the perceived importance of the procedures performed at each visit from a health maintenance point of view,

♦ the potential health benefits associated with treatment versus potential risks,

♦ the amount of discomfort produced by the study treatments or procedures performed,

♦ the amount of effort required of the patient to maintain the treatment regime,

♦ the number and type of side effects associated with treatment.

In recent times the problems of non-compliance in a clinical trial have been well illustrated in trials involving HIV/AIDS patients, where an atmosphere of rapidly alternating hopes and disappointments has added to the difficulties of keeping patients on a fixed long-term treatment schedule.

So what can be done to ensure maximal patient compliance? Aspects of the study design may help; the shorter the trial, for example, the more likely subjects are to comply with the intervention regimen. So a study started and completed in one day would have great advantages over longer trials. And studies in which the subjects are under close supervision, such as in-patient hospital-based trials, tend to have fewer problems of non-compliance. Reducing the amount of data being collected can only improve compliance—a good motto is 'collect less data from more people'.

Simplicity of intervention may also affect compliance, with single dose drug regimens usually being preferable to those requiring multiple doses. The interval between scheduled visits to hospital or clinic is also a factor to consider. Too long an interval between visits may lead to a steady fall in patient compliance due to lack of encouragement, while too short an interval may prove a nuisance and reduce cooperation.

Perhaps the most important factor in maintaining good subject compliance once a trial has begun is the attitude of the staff running the trial. Experienced investigators stay in close contact with the patients early after randomization to get patients involved and, later, to keep them interested when their initial enthusiasm may have worn off. On the other hand, uninterested or discourteous staff will lead to an uninterested patient population. Meinert (1986) lists a number of simple factors likely to enhance patient participation and interest; this list is reproduced here in Table 2.1.

Table 2.1 Factors and approaches that enhance patient interest and participation.

- Clinic staff who treat patients with courtesy and dignity and who take an interest in meeting their needs.
- Clinic located in pleasant physical surroundings and in a secure environment.
- Convenient access to parking for patients who drive, and to other modes of transportation for those who do not.
- Payment of parking and travel fees incurred by study patients.
- Payment of clinic registration fees and costs for procedures required in the trial.
- Special clinics in which patients are able to avoid the confusion and turmoil of a regular out-patient clinic.
- Scheduled appointments designed to minimize waiting time.
- Clinic hours designed for patient convenience.
- Written or telephone contacts between clinic visits.
- Remembering patients on special occasions, such as Christmas, birthday anniversaries, etc.
- Establishment of identity with the study through proper indoctrination and explanation of study procedures during the enrolment process; through procedures such as the use of special ID cards to identify the patient as a participant in the study, and by awarding certificates to recognize their contributions to the trial.

Source: Taken with permission of Oxford University Press from Meinert, 1986.

Monitoring compliance is a crucial part of many clinical trials, since according to Friedman, Furberg and DeMets (1985):

> ... the interpretation of study results will be influenced by knowledge of compliance with the intervention. To the extent that the control group is not truly a control group and the intervention group is not being treated as intended, group differences may be diluted, leading possibly to an underestimate of the therapeutic effect and an under-reporting of adverse effects.

Differential compliance to two equally effective regimens can also lead to possibly erroneous conclusions about the effect of intervention.

In some studies measuring compliance is relatively easy. For example, trials in which one group receives surgery and the other group does not. Most of the time, however, assessment of compliance is not so simple and can rarely be established perfectly. In drug trials one of the most commonly used methods of evaluating subject compliance is pill or capsule count. But the method is far from foolproof. Even when a subject returns the appropriate number of leftover pills at a scheduled visit, the question of whether the remaining pills were used according to the protocol remains largely unanswered. Good rapport with the subjects will encourage cooperation and lead to a more accurate pill count, although there is considerable evidence that shows that the method can be unreliable and potentially misleading (see, for example, Cramer *et al.*, 1988; Waterhouse *et al.*, 1993).

Laboratory determinations can also sometimes be used to monitor compliance to medications. Tests done on either blood or urine can detect the presence of active drugs or metabolites. For example, Hjalmarson *et al.* (1981) checked compliance with metroprobol therapy after myocardial infarction by using assays of metroprobol in urine. Several other approaches to monitoring compliance are described in Friedman, Furberg and De Mets (1985), and Senn (1997) mentions two recent technical developments that may be useful, namely:

◆ Electronic monitoring—pill dispensers with a built-in microchip which will log when the dispenser is opened,

◆ Low-dose, slow turnover chemical markers which can be added to treatment and then detected via blood-sampling.

The claim is often made that in published drug trials more than 90% of patients have been satisfactorily compliant with the protocol-specified dosing regimen. But Urquhart and DeKlerk (1998) suggest that these claims, based as they usually are, on count of returned dosing forms, which patients can easily manipulate, are exaggerated, and that data from the more reliable methods for measuring compliance mentioned above, contradict them.

Clinical trial investigators, particularly those dealing with psychiatric trials should not assume that patients take their medication regularly. Non-compliance may lead to the investigator transferring a patient to the alternative therapy or withdrawing the patient from the study altogether; often such decisions are taken out of the investigators' hands by the patient simply refusing to participate in the trial any further and thus becoming a trial dropout (see Chapter 5). When non-compliance manifests as dropout from a study, the connection with missing data is direct. In other circumstances manifestation of non-compliance is more complex and some response is observed, but a question remains about what would have been observed had compliance been achieved.

Non-compliance, leading either to receiving treatment other than that provided for by the results of randomization, or to dropping out of the trial altogether, has serious implications for the analysis of the data collected in a clinical trial, implications which will be taken up again in later chapters. (As well as being a problem in clinical trials, non-compliance is, of course, also a serious problem in the day-to-day treatment of many psychiatric patients, and several attempts have been made to improve this situation by introducing *compliance therapy*, a talking treatment based partly on motivational interviewing and cognitive behavioural therapy. The participant is invited to review their history of illness, symptoms and side-effects and consider the benefits and drawbacks of drug treatment. A report of a clinical trial of compliance therapy is given in Kemp *et al.*, 1996.)

2.6 Summary

According to Palmer (2002):

> Clinical trials are a composite of matters, ethical, practical, and theoretical. They have had a short but distinguished history, having rapidly become the accepted

norm for benchmarking medical progress and yielding the highest quality, single-study evidence for treatment efficacy. This is due to the fundamental and unique role of randomisation that allows cause-and-effect inferences to be made linking patients' treatment allocations and their subsequent health outcomes.

The randomized controlled clinical trial has, over the last fifty years, become one of the most important tools in medical research in general, and psychiatric research in particular. Indeed, according to the British statistician, Sir David Cox, the RCT is perhaps the outstanding contribution of statistics to twentieth (and twenty-first) century medical research. Clinical trials do, of course, have their limitations—they have, for example, a limited ability to test for safety since they only evaluate relatively small numbers of patients and they tend to exclude patients who are susceptible to complications. Nevertheless they remain the most powerful tool in the armoury of researchers seeking to find the best treatment for a particular condition.

Broad ethical arguments against clinical trials (patients should not be guinea pigs) are today largely recognized as misplaced and misguided, and most clinicians (including most psychiatrists) now have little difficulty in allowing their patients to take part in such trials, and likewise we hope that the informed patient will also understand the cogent reasons for agreeing to participate. Certainly clinical trials in psychiatry have become commonplace and it is doubtful that any modern day psychiatrist would comment on a trial as William Sargant did on the MRC's trial of the treatment of depressive illness less than 30 years ago:

> There is no psychiatric illness in which bedside knowledge and long clinical experience pays better dividends; and we are never going to learn how to treat depression properly from double-blind sampling in an MRC statistician's office.

Sargant was not allowed to have the last word however; Bradford Hill replied to his comments with typical good humour in his Heberden Oration of 1965:

> I am sure he [*Sargant*] is right on both counts. Unfortunately, as one of the patients in the bed, I feel more than a trifle depressed while-partly at my expense—he gains his knowledge and his long clinical experience. I would have hoped that the process of learning might be a little less long if it were supported by the experimental method and attitude of mind.

But amongst the growing number of psychiatric trials now taking place, a sizable minority continue to be plagued by poor design, inadequate data, and incorrect or misleading analysis with the result that even after many studies in some areas, little has really been learnt. We hope that the material presented in the remainder of this book will help to improve this situation.

Chapter 3

Design issues in clinical trials

3.1 Introduction

The first question to be addressed by anyone contemplating carrying out a clinical trial is whether it is appropriate to mount the trial at all? If previous trials have conclusively demonstrated the effectiveness (or lack of effectiveness) of a treatment, there is little point in investigating that treatment further. This may seem an obvious truism but it has not always been followed. Chalmers and Lau (1993), for example, looked at a series of randomized clinical trials of endoscopic treatment of bleeding peptic ulcer carried out from the 1980s to the 1990s. Combining the results from trials up to 1982 showed that the chances that endoscopic therapy was not reducing recurrent or continued bleeding, when compared to the standard therapy, were less than one in a thousand. Yet in the 25th published trial, carried out between 1989 and 1991, patients continued to be randomly assigned to a control group. Chalmers and Lau asked the question, 'If the authors of the later publications knew of the previous ones, how much proof did they require?' and posed the further question 'When is it no longer ethical to assign patients at random to a control group in a new definitive large trial?' Much the same point was made by Antman and colleagues in their now classic analysis of the time lag between when an ongoing meta analysis would have revealed that post myocardial infarction thrombolytic therapy saved lives, and its routine introduction into cardiological practice. This knowledge could have been available even before the mega trial of thrombolytic therapy was launched (Antman *et al.*, 1992).

Assuming an investigator is convinced that his or her proposed trial *is* necessary, they are faced with a considerable number of issues in both designing and organizing the trial. What is the best trial design to answer the specific question being addressed? How many subjects will I need to obtain a precise estimate of the treatment effect? How do I set about recruiting the required number and type of participants? Having recruited the patients, what is the most appropriate method of randomization? How do I measure how the subjects in the trial are performing?

How do I maintain blindness? Should I have rules about when or if to stop the trial before the end envisaged in the trial protocol? How do I ensure compliance, and what happens if I don't?

We shall address some of these questions in this chapter; others which are of particular importance for psychiatric trials such as how to measure outcome and the recruitment of patients with a specified diagnosis, will be left until Chapter 4.

3.2 Clinical trial designs

Although the fundamental aim of all clinical trials is essentially the same, that is to discover if one treatment is 'better' than an alternative, the trials can be arranged or designed in different ways to achieve this aim. In this section, we will examine the principal types of clinical trial design that are used in practice.

3.2.1 Parallel groups

The majority of clinical trials involve parallel treatment groups. In the simplest situation patients are randomized to one of two treatments under study. The word parallel indicates that the groups formed by randomization proceed through the trial side by side, with the only difference between them being the treatment administered (apart, of course, from possible baseline differences). The aim of parallel treatment design trials is for each participant to receive the assigned treatment and to have no exposure to any of the other treatments under study in the trial (except where this is deemed necessary in response to say a severe adverse event).

The parallel groups design trial is the easiest to manage and the easiest to analyse, although it does have some drawbacks, particularly in maintaining subjects in the control treatment condition, whatever it may be. Nevertheless, this design remains the simplest and most popular for clinical trials in all areas including psychiatry. Examples of the use of the parallel groups design can be found in almost all current issues of the major psychiatric journals; two recent ones are:

- Conley and Mahmoud (2001) describe a parallel groups study involving a comparison of risperidone and olanzapine in the treatment of schizophrenia.
- Bondareff et al. (2000) compare sertraline and nortriptyline in the treatment of major depressive disorder in later life.

3.2.2 Crossover trials

With a crossover design each participant in a trial receives two or more study treatments in a specified order. For example, in a two-period crossover design, each person receives each of two treatments (A and B) either in the order AB or BA; the order is usually chosen at random. So the trial would consist of two groups: the members of one having received the treatments in the order AB, and the members of the other in the order BA. Clearly such a design is only suitable for stable chronic conditions in which there is the limited objective of studying the patient's response to relatively short periods of therapy.

Crossover trials produce *within* participant comparisons, whereas parallel designs produce *between* participant comparisons. As each participant acts as his or her own control in crossover trials, they can produce statistically and clinically valid results with fewer participants than would be required with a parallel design. Furthermore, because patients are exposed to both treatments, some interesting data can often be gathered on patient preference. Sadly these advantages of a crossover design come at a considerable cost, namely the possibility of a *carryover effect*, caused by interference between the two treatments. The problem is that when we come to study the results from a given period of treatment for a given patient, the results may reflect not only the effect of the current treatment, but also the effect of the previous treatment. The disentangling of one effect from another may be extremely difficult. In an attempt to deal with this potential difficulty, crossover designs almost always include a 'wash out' interval between the times participants are receiving the two treatments. But one can never be sure this wash out period is effective, and it is also exceedingly difficult to arrange such an interval for anything other than a drug trial.

Crossover designs are dealt with in great detail in Senn (2001). An example of the use of the design in psychiatry is provided by the study of secretin for the treatment of autistic disorder reported by Owley *et al.* (2001). In this study 20 autistic subjects received either a secretin or placebo infusion at baseline and the other substance at week four. The study found no evidence for the efficacy of secretin in the treatment of autistic disorder.

3.2.3   Factorial designs

The majority of clinical trials have focused on treatments used separately from each other, although this does not match up with clinical practice where it is rarely sufficient to consider only a single treatment for a condition. Questions about the effects of *combinations* of treatments may, consequently, often be of interest but cannot be answered by the simple parallel groups design or the crossover design. Instead a factorial design is used in which several treatments are not only evaluated separately, but also in combination and against a control. A classic factorial design for two treatments A and B would consist of randomizing prospective participants to each of the four cells of the following table:

Treatment A and Placebo A	Treatment B and Placebo B
Treatment A and Treatment B	Placebo A and Placebo B

Factorial designs are of most use when possible *interactions* between therapeutic combinations are of *primary* interest (see Holtzman *et al.*, 1987; Berry, 1990). An interaction occurs when the effect of a combination of treatments differs from the sum of the individual effects of each treatment. Factorial designs are less useful if estimation of simple treatment effects is required, unless interactions between the various treatments can be ruled out *a priori*; if they cannot, then factorial designs will require larger sample sizes to achieve the same power as a parallel groups design. Lubsen and Pocock (1994) suggest that the possibility of being able to dismiss interactions between treatments *a priori* is small.

An example of a factorial trial is a study that looked at how to improve compliance with antidepressant medication in primary care. There were two interventions—either a leaflet giving information or a session of counselling, both or neither. The results showed that counselling alone improved compliance (Peveler *et al.*, 1999).

3.2.4 Patient preference trials

In Chapter 2, we stressed that the ethical pre-requisite for undertaking a clinical trial is that the researcher is in a state of equipoise—not knowing which of the two or more options under study is the best treatment for his or her patient. In the same chapter we also argued that equipoise is the rule, rather than the exception, for many clinical interventions and situations in psychiatry. However, even when a sober assessment suggests that we genuinely do not know which is the best treatment to advice for a patient, and thus a state of equipoise exists, this may not be a view shared by the patients themselves. Patients as well as clinicians can have treatment preferences, preferences that may persist even if a clinician informs them that there really is no sound evidence favouring one treatment over another. It is likely, for example, that many psychiatric patients will have firm views about the role of drugs for treating mental conditions, since opinion surveys regularly show that a substantial proportion of the population remain opposed to the use of antidepressants for mental disorders, despite the evidence supporting their efficacy. Certainly clinical trial investigators frequently report difficulties in randomizing patients to trials in which drugs are compared with psychotherapies, since many patients make it clear that irrespective of the evidence for equipoise proposed by the researcher, they have a preference for one intervention over the other. In a randomized trial, particularly if the clinician is blind to treatment assignment, patient preference may be a more important issue than clinician preference.

If eligible individuals refuse to participate in a trial, either because they have a strong preference for one particular intervention (if there are several active interventions available) or because they do not want to receive a placebo, and other eligible individuals decide to participate in a trial despite having a clear preference for one of the study interventions, what might be the effect on the results? The important question that needs to be addressed is, are the outcomes of these individuals, whether they enter the trial or not, different from those participants who do not have strong preferences?

Clearly some patient preferences definitely *do* influence outcome—a preference for drugs over psychotherapy may be related to factors such as age, gender, socio-economic status, previous illness and so on, all of which are known confounders of prognosis, and thus influence outcome. These can be studied, adjusted for, and of course will largely be dealt with by randomization.

But is there a more subtle, psychological or suggestive effect of patient preference? Some authors (Brewin and Bradley, 1989, for example) believe there is, and that it is closely related, but not synonymous with, the better-known placebo effect. Given, however that the size and even existence of the latter remains uncertain (Gotzsche and Lange, 1991), it is not surprising that neither clinicians nor other clinical trial investigators can agree on the importance of patient preference (McPherson *et al.*, 1997). If patient preference *is* a problem, it is likely to be particularly acute in many psychiatric trials, for example any trial involving a talking therapy, since the trial cannot be double blind.

An example of a clinical trial in which patient preference was allowed is that carried out by King and colleagues at the Royal Free Hospital in London (Ward *et al.*, 2000). This was a pragmatic trial (see Chapters 2 and 6) that sought to compare non-directive counselling, CBT and usual GP care. The problem was that many patients already had views about which would work for them, even if there was no sound scientific evidence for their views. Patients were therefore allowed to opt for any of the three treatments if they had a strong wish to do so—most chose CBT. In fact it was even more complex than that, since it turned out that actually the real patient preference was to avoid usual care from the GP, but most did not mind which of the two psychological therapies they should receive. The result was a complex randomization scheme, in which a three-way randomization was made between the three arms of the trial, with a two-way randomization between CBT and counselling—in effect a double patient preference trial.

Although this was a heroic effort to try and deliver a trial that came closest to clinical reality, the result was, as one might expect, a trial that remains difficult to interpret. In fact, the principle finding was that the two psychological treatments group were superior to usual care, but were equivalent themselves. Finally, at the end of the trial, all three groups were equally effective. Perhaps this was fortunate since problems could have arisen if at the end of the day one group had been declared clearly superior to the others; the latter finding would, no doubt, have been greeted with accusations of selection bias that would have been difficult to refute.

The critical, and to our mind insuperable, problem with patient preference trials is that they violate the principle of randomization. When all is said and done, those in the patient preference arm have not been randomly allocated. Any result in that arm is likely to be influenced by selection bias and confounding, and thus any observed treatment effect becomes difficult to interpret unambiguously. From a statistical viewpoint, patient preference designs appear to be a blind alley. A statistical analysis strategy that highlights the effects of preferences and thus leads to a clearer understanding of what we need to concentrate on in the interpretation of results is described in Dunn *et al.* (2003).

3.2.5 Randomization prior to consent—the 'Zelen' design

Another study design that differs from the standard parallel group design is known as *Zelen's design*; here prospective participants for the trial are randomized to one of the study treatments *prior* to giving their consent to take part in the trial.

Those who are allocated to receive the standard treatment or intervention are given this treatment but are not told they are part of a trial, although they may be asked for consent to follow up. The individuals who are randomized to receiving the experimental treatment are then approached, told they are part of a trial and offered the new treatment. If they decline to take part in the trial, they are then given the standard treatment but are analysed as if they had received the new treatment. Zelen's design is illustrated in Fig. 3.1.

Zelen's design has a number of advantages. It can, for example, make the act of recruitment and randomization simpler and more effective by avoiding the need to obtain full consent from those patients who receive the control condition, with which they might have been disappointed, had they had their hopes raised of receiving the new intervention. Of course, trials should only be done when the investigator is convinced there is a state of equipoise, and that there is no evidence that one treatment is better than the other, but in reality many patients (and of course investigators) may not see it that way. By improving recruitment, Zelen's design can also reduce selection bias, and reduce drop out. The latter is the principal reason why such a design was chosen as the most appropriate approach for a Dutch study of heroin provision for chronic heroin addicts (Schellings *et al.*, 1999).

Further advantages of Zelen's design are that almost all eligible individuals are included in the trial and the design does allow the true treatment effect to be estimated. The specific disadvantages of this type of design are that trials that use it have to be open trials and the statistical power of the study may be adversely affected if a large number of the available participants choose to have the standard treatment, which also introduces probable bias.

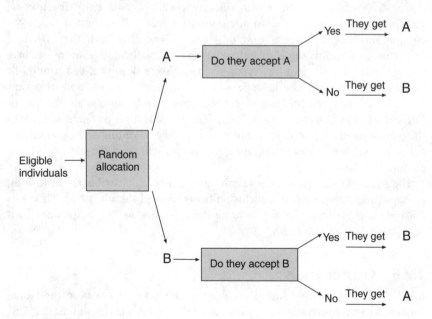

Fig. 3.1 Diagram showing Zelen's design.

An example of the use of Zelen's design is a study in which patients with chronic benign headache referred to a neurologist are randomly allocated to being offered an MRI scan or not (Howard *et al.*, submitted). The aim of the trial is to assess whether or not provision of an unnecessary investigation (any patient in whom the neurologist actually wishes to perform a scan, a rare event, obviously not randomized) does indeed provide reassurance and a reduction in anxiety, as many neurologists believe, or alternatively has the opposite effect, as many psychiatrists believe. The Zelen design was chosen because it would severely bias the study if those who are not going to receive a scan that they do not need were informed of the purpose of the study. There appeared to be no ethical problems with the study, since those randomized to the control arm have not had any change whatsoever in their care, nor have they been deprived of an intervention that they might need. Certainly both the ethics committee that considered the study design and the editors of the journal to which the report was submitted agreed that the Zelen design chosen for investigation was acceptable. The trial found that giving patients with chronic headache an MRI when not clinically indicated did indeed reduce symptoms and was also cost-effective—one up to the neurologists!

Another example of the use of a Zelen design is provided by a clinical trial that examined the effect of adding a family worker to the care of stroke patients (Dennis, 1997). This was published in the *British Medical Journal* (BMJ), and triggered a lively debate about the ethics of not obtaining consent before randomizing subjects (Dennis, 1997). Whilst there was a view from an ethicist that this practice could never be justified in any circumstances, the authors provided a vigorous defence, saying that this was ethical, as well as producing better science, a view with which we and others concur (Schellings *et al.*, 1999; Truog *et al.*, 1999). It is also the case that non-consented research is permitted in certain circumstances by the Declaration of Helsinki, and that both the FDA and Department of Health and Human Services in the United States allow researchers to waive informed consent for certain research under clearly defined conditions (such as to allow critically ill patients access to new therapies, and to permit research in such circumstances—echoed, albeit ambiguously, in the recent European Union Directive, Visser, 2001). The 'CRASH' trial, a trial of steroids in the management of severe head injury, is currently recruiting and randomizing many thousands of patients without informed consent from the participants for obvious reasons (see Table 3.1).

The ethics of non-consented research was extensively debated in the BMJ, with, perhaps predictably, no firm conclusion being reached (Smith, 1997). This does illustrate one particular hazard of using the Zelen design—the results obtained may prove difficult to publish.

3.2.6 Cluster trials

In all the discussions of clinical trials up to this point it has been individual patients who have been randomized to one of the treatment arms of the trial. This is the most common situation in clinical trial work, but there are situations where

Table 3.1 Circumstances in which non-consented randomization might be considered (from Truog et al., 1999).

◆ Treatments offered within the trial would be available outside the trial anyway without the specific informed consent of the patient.

◆ Each intervention should be of similar risk.

◆ Genuine clinical equipoise must exist between the interventions.

◆ No reasonable person could be expected to have a strong preference for one treatment over the other.

◆ Full ethical scrutiny has taken place.

◆ Critically ill patients from whom it is impossible to obtain consent, but who might as a group benefit from the results of research.

---

randomization of individuals is simply not possible and others where it is not desirable. In such cases, groups or clusters of individuals may become the unit of randomization. For example, patients attending a particular therapist or clinical practice, or a single screening centre and so on might have to be randomized as a group rather than as individuals. And when a group of individuals so interact with each other that they are not truly independent it may be better to randomize them together rather than separately; an example would be a trial involving members of a number of army units where it is inevitable that individuals within units will exchange stories and swop information, in particular about any treatment they are receiving and its perceived effects.

Trials in which intact social units, or clusters of individuals, rather than individuals themselves, are randomized to different intervention groups are known as cluster randomization or group randomization trials. Such trials are becoming increasingly popular in the evaluation of non-therapeutic interventions, including lifestyle modification, educational programmes and innovations in the provision of health care. The units of randomization in such trials range from households or families to hospital wards, classrooms and medical practices; more unusual cluster randomization studies have involved athletic teams (Walsh et al., 1999), tribes (Glasgow et al., 1995), religious institutions (Lancaster et al., 1997) and sex establishments (Fontanet et al., 1998).

Superficially randomizing clusters of individuals sounds most alluring—at the metaphorical toss of a single coin a large numbers of subjects have been recruited to the trial, all in one go. But, as always, things are not so simple as they may appear. The problem is that, in a statistical sense at least, cluster allocation schemes are less efficient than randomizing individuals. The loss of efficiency arises because the response of individuals in an intact cluster tend to be more similar than the responses of individuals in different clusters—there is, essentially, a reduction in the effective sample size for the trial, the effect increasing with an increase in *intracluster correlation coefficient*, a measure of the lack of independence of the members of a cluster. The result is a loss of precision in estimating the effect of the intervention.

But although such trials are less efficient relative to individual randomization, they may still be the design of choice when the individuals to be treated arise naturally in groups, or there is a need to minimize experimental contamination, or in some cases for ethical reasons. An example of a cluster randomization trial used for both ethical reasons and to avoid contamination is provided by the study reported in Sommer *et al.* (1986). The aim of the investigation was to evaluate the effect of vitamin A supplementation on childhood mortality. In the trial, 450 villages in Indonesia were randomly assigned either to participate in vitamin A supplementation or to serve as a control. Cluster randomization was adopted because it was 'not considered politically feasible' to randomize individuals. It may also be noted that randomization of intact villages avoided the contamination that could have arisen if individuals within a village randomly assigned to different interventions were to share the same medication.

A good example of a psychiatric cluster randomized trial is the Hampshire Depression Project (Thompson *et al.*, 2000), which used a cluster randomized design to repeat at the time seminal observation of Gotz on the Danish island of Bornholm. Gotz reported a non-randomized intervention in which the island's GPs were given an education package to improve the recognition and management of depression. This intervention package apparently led to a decrease in the suicide rate. Reducing the suicide rate is the Holy Grail of public health physicians/psychiatrists, so this study was widely cited and became incorporated into policy in, for example, this country.

Thompson and colleagues at the University of Southampton performed a cluster randomized trial to replicate the intervention. Randomization took place at the practice level, since otherwise there would have been contamination between partners in the practice, if one had received the intervention and the other had not, and patients, since they could attend one GP who had received the training, and then another who had not. The trial failed to demonstrate any effect on patient outcomes.

The analysis of cluster randomization trials is generally more complex than for those in which individuals are the unit of randomization, since there is a need to account for the lack of independence of the responses given by the members of the same cluster. A detailed account of how to analyse such trials is given in Donner and Klar (2000) and other useful references are Kerry and Bland (1998); Piaggio *et al.*, (2001).

3.2.7 Multicentre trials

The usual single centre trial remains, for the present, the back bone of psychiatric research (Warlow, 1990). But such trials are limited when it comes to trying to achieve the aim of a large simple trial (see Chapter 8) since they will be unable to recruit enough participants in a time period short enough to make the trial viable. Instead recruitment will need to involve several centres (for example, clinics, hospitals, etc.) along with a common treatment and data collection protocol and a central point to receive and process study data. Such *multicentre trials* offer a number of

Multicentre trial organization

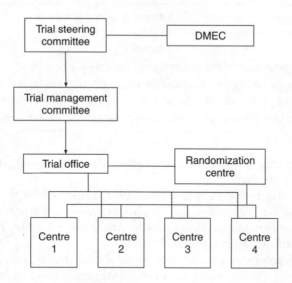

Fig. 3.2 Multicentre trial organization.

advantages over the single centre study, the most obvious being the increase in patient accrual, both in scale and speed. But there are also other advantages, related to the wider range of patients that will be included in the trial, thus increasing the likely generalizability and dissemination of the results when they become available. With a multicentre trial it will be harder to argue that the results are only related to a small group of, by implication atypical, patients. Multicentre trials can also foster other collaborations, both national and international.

Of course, there is no such thing as a free lunch, and multicentre trials pose their own problems, some obvious, some less so. The most obvious relates to the increased problems of co-ordination and organization (see Fig. 3.2 for a summary of how such trials need to be organized). Multicentre trials need the tightest attention to detail and co-ordination, with the setting up of an efficient central trial office, and employment of an equally efficient and effective trial co-ordinator. Ensuring good quality control and reliability across the centres is vital, and will require frequent meetings and visits.

A further possible complication with a multicentre trial arises at the analysis stage, which must now take into account the possible heterogeneity introduced by the different centres. It is likely, for example, that the true treatment effect will not be identical at each centre. Consequently there may be some degree of treatment-by-centre interaction and various methods have been suggested for dealing with this possibility. Details are available in Jones *et al.* (1998), Gould (1998) and Senn (1998) and an example is provided in Chapter 6. Having said that, we note the comment of a number of experienced multicentre triallists that adjusting for centre 'probably makes no difference but helps to confirm a primary unadjusted

Table 3.2 Potential problems with multicentre trials.

◆ The planning and administration of any multicentre trial is considerably more complex than in a single centre.

◆ Multicentre trials are very expensive to run.

◆ Ensuring that all centres follow the study protocol may be difficult.

◆ Consistency of measurements across centres needs very careful attention.

◆ Motivating all participants in a large multicentre trial may be difficult.

◆ Lack of clear leadership may lead to a degradation in the quality of a multicentre trial.

---

analysis' (Assmann *et al.*, 2000). In other words it is a useful, and probably obligatory, quality check.

There are also problems with measurement, particularly if the sites are in different countries when there may be obvious language difficulties. Leese and colleagues describe the problems of achieving good reliability in measuring outcomes in this situation (Leese *et al.*, 2001).

Recommendations over the appropriate number of centres needed in a multicentre trial vary. On the one hand, rate of patient acquisition may be completely inadequate when dealing with a small number of centres, but with a larger number (20 or more) potential practical problems (see Table 3.2) may quickly outweigh benefits. Warlow, who has run more multicentre trials than most, provides a helpful discussion of the problems and pitfalls (Warlow, 1990).

3.3　Methods of randomization

Randomization was introduced in Chapter 2 as an elegant way of allocating participants to different treatments in a clinical trial that avoided selection bias, provided a sound basis for the estimation of the treatment effect and dealt directly with the problem of bias from potential confounders by distributing them randomly between the different treatments. It would seem that, in principle at least, randomization would be simplicity itself, involving nothing more than the toss of a fair coin. In practice however things are a little more complicated.

3.3.1　Complete randomization

Complete randomization (also often known as *simple randomization*) is simple coin tossing, although the flip of a coin is generally replaced in practice with the use of a table of random numbers or, more usually, a computer-based random number generator. In essence though the result is that a patient is allocated to say treatment A if a 'head' appears and to treatment B if the 'coin' shows a 'tail'. Each random allocation is by definition random, and is entirely independent of any preceding or subsequent allocation-treatment assignments are independent. The power of this method is that each treatment assignment is totally unpredictable. Consequently there can be no selection bias with complete randomization, since it is equally likely to guess the next treatment assignment correctly or incorrectly.

Unfortunately there is a disadvantage to complete randomization that makes it unattractive in practice; there is considerable potential for an imbalance in the number of patients allocated to each treatment, particularly when the trial is relatively small (as many trials in psychiatry are). Complete randomization is no guarantee of equal sized groups. If say 60 patients are to be randomly allocated between two treatments it is very unlikely that complete randomization will result in 30 in each group (Schultz and Grimes 2002); and when randomizing 50 patients to two treatments using this approach there is about a 5% probability of ending up with an imbalance between the groups of 14 patients or worse (Rosenberger and Lachin, 2002).

So with complete randomization there is a non-negligible probability of some imbalances between treatment groups. Such imbalances may be a source of concern for many investigators from a 'cosmetic' point of view, but the more important question is whether they will invalidate the statistical properties of the study? The answer appears to be that they will not. Whatever the imbalance the estimate of the treatment effect will remain unbiased, although the precision of the estimator will decrease but only slightly for moderate imbalances; and the power associated with the study will decrease only slowly in the move away from equal sized groups where it is at its greatest (See Pocock, 1983; Rosenberger and Lachin, 2002).

But despite the seeming lack of any dire statistical consequences resulting from an imbalance produced by complete randomization, investigators designing clinical trials will often still hanker after equal sized groups. The reason is that very uneven treatment group sizes can cause problems in the administration or even financing of a trial, particularly if the treatment under investigation is a psychological one, or a complex health intervention that may be subjected to limited resources. Consequently a number of *restricted* randomization methods have been developed, that ensure similar numbers in each treatment group throughout the trial. The most commonly used of these procedures is *blocked randomization*. (It should perhaps be mentioned here that, under certain conditions, unequal group sizes may be a sensible design requirement. Arranging to allocate a larger number of patients to a new treatment than to the standard treatment, for example, may be warranted by the need for fuller information about the general characteristics of the new treatment.)

3.3.2 Blocked randomization

This method, also known as *permuted block randomization*, guarantees that at no time during randomization will the imbalance be large and that at certain points the number of subjects in each group will be equal. The essential feature of this approach is that *blocks* of a particular number of patients are considered and a different random ordering of treatments assigned in each block; the process is repeated for consecutive blocks of patients until all have been randomized. For example, with two treatments (A and B), the investigator may want to ensure that after every sixth randomized subject, the number of subjects in each treatment group is equal. Then a block of size six would be used and the process would randomize the order in which three As and three Bs are assigned for every consecutive group of six subjects entering the trial. There are 20 possible sequences of three As and three Bs and one of these is chosen at random and the six subjects are assigned accordingly. The process is repeated as many times as possible. When six patients are enrolled, the numerical balance between treatment A and treatment B is equal and the equality is maintained with the enrollment of the 12th, 18th patient and so on.

Friedman *et al.* (1985) suggest an alternative method of blocked randomization in which random numbers between 0 and 1 are generated for each of the assignments within a block, and the assignment order then determined by the ranking of these numbers. For example, with a block of size six in the two-treatment situation we might have:

Assignment	Random number
A	0.112
A	0.675
A	0.321
B	0.018
B	0.991
B	0.423

This leads to the assignment order BAABAB.

In trials that are not double-blind, one potential problem with blocked randomization is that at the end of each block, alert clinicians can begin to guess the next allocation by noting the pattern of past assignments. Should the clinician become aware that the two groups are equal in size after every, for example, four participants, then it is not difficult to start influencing the allocation (Schultz and Grimes, 2002). The smaller the block size the greater is the risk of the randomization becoming predictable. For this reason repeated blocks of size two should *not* be used. One common solution is to insist that clinicians do not know the block size or even to randomly vary the block sizes themselves, which makes it very difficult to determine the next assignment in a series.

The great advantage of blocking is that balance between the number of subjects is guaranteed during the course of the randomization. The number in each group will never differ by more than $b/2$ where b is the size of the block. This can be important for two reasons. First if enrollment in a trial takes place slowly over a period of months or even years, the type of patient recruited for the study may change during the entry period (temporal changes in severity of illness, for example, are not uncommon), and blocking will produce more comparable groups. A second advantage of blocking is that if the trial should be terminated before enrollment is completed because of the results of some form of *interim analysis* (see later in this chapter), balance will exist in terms of number of subjects randomized to each group.

Strictly speaking, the statistical analysis of a trial in which blocked randomization is used needs to take into account the blocking procedure. In practice, however, there is some consensus that the complexities introduced are not worth the minimal extra gain in power (Wittes, 2001).

3.3.3 Stratified randomization

As mentioned in Chapter 2, one of the objectives in randomizing patients to treatment groups is to achieve between group comparability on certain relevant patient characteristics usually known as *prognostic factors*. Measured prior to randomization, these are factors that it is thought likely will correlate with subsequent patient response or outcome. For example, if it is known that educated patients are more likely to respond to a particular psychotherapy than the less educated, then one would want levels of education to be reasonably comparable between the groups, otherwise that might be an alternative explanation for why one group improved and the other did not.

Simple randomization tends to produce groups that are, on average, similar in their entry characteristics, both known and unknown. The larger a trial is, the less chance there will be of any serious non-comparability of treatment groups, but for a small study (and in psychiatry sample size is not always what it should be) there is no guarantee that all baseline characteristics will be similar in the two groups. If prognostic factors are not evenly distributed between treatment groups it may give the investigator cause for concern. If so the solution may be to use *stratified randomization* which is a procedure that helps achieve comparability between the study groups for a chosen set of prognostic factors. According to Pocock (1983), the method is rather like an insurance policy in that its primary aim is to guard against the unlikely event of the treatment groups ending up with some major difference in patient characteristics. The method is frequently performed in multicentre trials, since despite every effort by the investigators, differences between centres are the rule rather than the exception.

The first issue to be considered when contemplating stratified randomization is which prognostic factors should be considered. Experience of earlier trials may be useful here. When several prognostic factors are to be considered, a stratum for randomization is formed by selecting one subgroup from each of them (continuous variables such as age are divided into groups of some convenient range). Since the total number of strata is, therefore, the product of the number of subgroups in each factor, the number of strata increases rapidly as factors are added and the levels within factors are refined. Consequently only the most important variables should be chosen and the number kept to a minimum.

Within each stratum, the randomization process itself could be simple randomization, but in practice most clinical trials will use some blocked randomization approach. As an example, suppose that an investigator wishes to stratify on age and sex, and to use a block size of four. First age is divided into a number of categories, say 40–49, 50–59 and 60–69. The design thus has 3 × 2 strata, and the randomization might be:

Strata	Age	Sex	Group assignment
1	40–49	Male	ABBA BABA . . .
2	40–49	Female	
3	50–59	Male	
4	50–59	Female	
5	60–69	Male	
6	60–69	Female	

Patients between 40 and 49 years of age and male would be assigned to treatment groups A and B in the sequences ABBA BABA. . . . Similarly random sequences would appear in the other strata.

Although the main argument for stratified randomization is that of making the treatment groups comparable with respect to specific prognostic factors, it may also lead to increased power if the stratification is taken into account in the analysis, by reducing variability in group comparisons. Such reduction allows a study of a given size to detect smaller group differences in outcome measures or to detect a specified difference with fewer subjects.

The disadvantage of stratification is its complexity. As the technical requirements of the chosen randomization process increase, so do the chances of error. The costs of the trial also increase, and there is always the chance that some strata will have insufficient numbers, thus reducing power. The general advice if stratified randomization is to be used is to keep it simple. Only stratify, for example, on variables that are easy to measure such as gender or age (assuming these are considered predictive of outcome).

Stratified randomization is of most relevance in small trials, but even here it may not be profitable if there is uncertainty over the importance or reliability of prognostic factors or if the trial has a limited organization that might not cope well with complex randomization procedures. In many cases it may be more useful to employ a *stratified analysis* (*subgroup analysis*) or *analysis of covariance* to adjust for prognostic factors when assessing treatment differences (see Chapter 5).

3.3.4 Minimization method

A further approach to achieving balance between treatment groups on selected prognostic factors is to use an *adaptive randomization procedure* in which the chance of allocating a new patient to a particular treatment is adjusted according to any existing imbalances in the baseline characteristics of the groups. For example, if sex is a prognostic factor and one treatment group has more women than men, the allocation scheme is such that the next few male patients are more likely to be randomized into the group that currently has less men. This method is often referred to as *minimization* because imbalances in the distribution of prognostic factors are minimized.

In general the method is applied in situations involving several prognostic factors and patient allocation is then based on the aim of balancing the marginal treatment totals for each level of each factor. As an example of the application of minimization, imagine a clinical trial comparing a new treatment of depression (A) with the standard treatment (B). Table 3.2 shows 40 patients already allocated to the two treatments categorized by four prognostic factors. Suppose the next patient to be allocated is less than 40 years old, has a current episode of depression that has lasted longer than six months, is female and is currently taking other antidepressant drugs. Then, for each treatment, the numbers of patients in the corresponding four rows of Table 3.3 are added to give:

Sum for A = 16 + 18 + 20 + 15 = 69
Sum for B = 15 + 16 + 22 + 14 = 67

Minimization requires the new patient to be allocated to the treatment with the smallest marginal total, in this case treatment A. If the sums for A and B are equal, then simple randomization is used to allocate the patient.

The aim of minimization is to balance the distribution of specific characteristics within the treatment groups, but to do so efficiently. Although minimization is a largely non-random method of treatment allocation, Scott *et al.* (2002) find evidence that it is highly effective and recommend its wider adoption in the conduct of clinical trials.

Blocking, stratified randomization and minimization all have their part to play in allocating patients to treatments in some clinical trials. But as the sample size used in a trial increases to a respectable value (sample size estimation will be considered in Section 3.5) it is unlikely that the investigator will need to consider any other randomization scheme than complete randomization. Once the overall sample size has reached around 200, most authorities advise that stratification and so on becomes unnecessary, and simple randomization will be sufficient to minimize chance biases (Pocock, 1985). Simple randomization, properly performed, has the added powerful advantage of being impossible to predict.

Table 3.3 Treatment assignments by four prognostic factors for 60 patients in a trial for a new treatment of depression.

Factor	Level	A	B
Age	Less than 40	16	15
	Greater than 40	14	15
Length of current episode	Less than 6 months	12	14
	Greater than 6 months	18	16
Sex	Male	10	8
	Female	20	22
Currently taking other anti-depressants?	Yes	15	14
	No	15	16

3.4 Methods of masking treatments

In Chapter 2 we showed that crucial to the integrity of a trial is good allocation concealment—ensuring that the investigators carrying out the trial have no possibility whatsoever of influencing who receives what intervention. There are various ways in which this can be achieved in practice—see Table 3.4—bearing in mind that the bottom line remains that the person who generates the randomization sequence must not in any circumstances be the person who decides who enters the trial. It will be clear that central computerized randomization carried out by a third party, but on an individual basis (i.e. not providing lists of future assignments to the investigators) is the counsel of perfection, and in this electronic age is not difficult to arrange. Many clinical trial support services, both commercial and academic, offer such a service.

3.5 The size of a clinical trial

One of the most frequent questions faced by a statistician dealing with investigators planning a clinical trial is 'how many participants do I need to recruit to each treatment group?' Answering the question requires consideration of a number of factors, for example, the amount of time available for the trial, the likely ease or difficulty in recruiting the type of patient required, and the possible financial constraints that may be involved. But the statistician may, initially at least, largely ignore these important aspects of the problem and apply a statistical procedure for calculating sample size that involves the following:

- Identifying the response variable of most interest.
- Specifying the appropriate statistical test to be used in the analysis of the chosen response.

Table 3.4 Different methods of allocation concealment (taken with permission of Elsevier from Schultz and Grimes, 2002, *Lancet*).

Allocation concealment system	Additional elements improving security
Sequentially numbered, opaque sealed envelopes (SNOSE)	Envelopes are opened only after the participant's name is written on the envelope. Within the envelope is some form of pressure sensitive carbon paper. The envelope is impermeable to light
Sequentially numbered containers	All the containers look the same, and cannot be tampered with
Pharmacy controlled	Clear documentation that the pharmacy is experienced in randomization, and clear documentation of exactly what randomizations scheme is being used
Central randomization	Ensure that the patient is enrolled in the trial and registered before the request is made for randomization

- Setting the size of the Type I error, that is, the significance level.
- Assessing the likely variance of the response variable.
- Agreeing with the investigators on the *power* they would like to achieve; for those readers who have forgotten (or perhaps never knew), the power of a statistical test is its probability of rejecting the null hypothesis when it is false.
- Obtaining from the investigators a size of treatment effect that is of clinical importance, that is, a treatment difference that the investigators would not like to miss being able to declare to be statistically significant.

So the investigators need to specify the size of the treatment difference considered clinically relevant (that is, important to detect) and with what degree of certainty, that is, with what power, it should be detected. Given such information the calculation of the corresponding sample size is often relatively straightforward, although the details will depend on the type of response variable and the type of test involved (see below for an example). In general terms the sample size will increase as the variability of the response variable increases and decrease as the chosen clinically relevant treatment effect increases. In addition the sample size will need to be larger to achieve a greater power and/or a more stringent significance level.

As an example of the calculations involved in sample size determination consider a trial involving the comparison of two treatments for anorexia nervosa. Anorexic women are to be randomly assigned to each treatment and the gain in weight in kilograms after three months is to be used as the outcome measure. From previous experience gained in similar trials it is known that the standard deviation (σ) of weight gain is likely to be about 4 kg. The investigator feels that a difference in weight gain of 1 kg (Δ) would be of clinical importance, and wishes to have a power of 90% when the appropriate two-sided test is used with significance level of 0.05 (α). The formula for calculating the number of women required in each treatment group (n) is

$$n = \frac{2(Z_{\alpha/2} + Z_\beta)^2 \sigma^2}{\Delta^2} \tag{3.1}$$

where β is 1-Power, and

- $Z_{\alpha/2}$ is the value of the normal distribution that cuts off an upper tail probability of $\alpha/2$. So for $\alpha = 0.05$, $Z_{\alpha/2} = 1.96$.
- Z_β is the value of the normal distribution that cuts off an upper tail probability of β. So for a power of 0.90, $\beta = 0.10$ and $Z_\beta = 1.28$.

So for the anorexia trial

$$n = \frac{2 \times (1.96 + 1.28)^2 \times 4^2}{1} = 336 \text{ women per treatment group.}$$

The example given above is clearly simplistic in the context of most psychiatric clinical trials, in which measurements of the response variable are likely to be made at several different time points, during which time some patients may dropout of the trial (see Chapter 6 for a discussion of such *longitudinal data* and the dropout problem).

Fortunately the last decade or so has produced a large volume of methodology useful in planning the size of randomized clinical trials with a variety of different types of outcome measures and with the complications outlined; some examples are to be found in Lee (1983), McHugh and Lee (1984), Schoenfield (1983), Sich (1987), Witters and Wallenstein (1987) and Spiegelhalter *et al.* (1994). In many cases tables are available which enable the required sample size for chosen power, significance level, effect size and so on to be simply read off. Increasingly these are being replaced by computer software for determining sample size for many standard and non-standard designs and outcome measures (see Appendix C).

An obvious danger with the sample size determination procedure mapped out above is that investigators (and, in some cases, even their statisticians) may occasionally be led to specify an effect size that is unrealistically extreme (what Senn, 1997, has described with his usual candor as 'a cynically relevant difference') so that the calculated sample size looks feasible in terms of possible pressing temporal and financial constraints. Such a possibility may be what led Senn (1997) to describe power calculations as 'a guess masquerading as mathematics' and Pocock (1996) to comment that they are 'a game that can produce any number you wish with manipulative juggling of the parameter values'. Statisticians advising on clinical trials need to be active in estimating the degree of difference that can be realistically expected for a clinical trial based on previous studies of a particular disease or, when such information is lacking, perhaps based on subjective opinions of investigators and physicians *not* involved in the proposed trial.

Getting the sample size right in a clinical trial is generally believed to be critical; indeed according to Simon (1991):

> An effective clinical trial must ask an important question and provide a reliable answer. A major determinant of the reliability of the answer is the sample size of the trial. Trials of inadequate size may cause contradictory and erroneous results and thereby lead to an inappropriate treatment of patients. They also divert limited resources from useful applications and cheat the patients who participated in what they thought was important clinical research. Sample size planning is, therefore, a key component of clinical trial methodology.

Certainly many clinical trial investigators would (and have) argued that trials with 'inadequate' sample size are, in a very real sense, unethical in that they require patients to accept the risks of treatment, however small, without any chance of benefit to them or future patients. Freiman *et al.* (1978), for example, reviewed 71 'negative' randomized clinical trials, that is trials in which the observed differences between the proposed and control treatments were not large enough to satisfy a specified 'significance' level (the risk of a type I error) and the results were declared to be 'not statistically significant'. Analysis of these clinical studies indicated that the investigators often worked with numbers of enrolled patients too small to offer a reasonable chance of avoiding the opposing mistake, a type II error (accepting the null hypothesis when it is false). Fifty of the trials had a greater than 10% risk of missing a substantial difference (true treatment difference of 50%) in treatment outcome. The reviewers warned that many treatments labelled as 'not different from control' had not received a critical test because the trials had insufficient power to do the job intended. Freiman *et al.*'s examples clearly illustrate the truth in that memorable phrase of Altman and Bland, 'absence of evidence is not evidence of absence'.

This concern about patient numbers in many clinical trials being too small is echoed by Pocock (1996), who sees the problem as 'a general phenomena whose full implications for restricting therapeutic progress are not widely appreciated'. In the same article Pocock continues:

> The fact is that trials with truly modest treatment effects will achieve statistical significance only if random variation conveniently exaggerated these effects. The chances of publication and reader interest are much greater if the results of the trial are statistically significant. Hence the current obsession with significance testing combined with the inadequate size of many trials means that publications on clinical trials for many treatments are likely to be biased towards an exaggeration of therapeutic effect, even if the trials are unbiased in all other respects.

The primary purpose in making a trial as large as possible is to maximize the chance of detecting a treatment effect, particularly if that effect is not very big, and to provide a precise estimate of the size of the treatment effect. A large trial may also allow a few sensible and pre-defined sub-group analyses to try to assess for whom the treatment works best (see Chapter 5). The case against trials with inadequate numbers of subjects appears strong but as Senn (1997) points out, sometimes only a small trial is possible. And misinterpreting a non-significant effect as an indication that a treatment effect is not effective rather than as a failure to *prove* that it is effective, suggests trying to improve medical education rather than totally abandoning small trials. In addition with the growing use of *systematic reviews* and *meta-analysis*, topics to be discussed in Chapter 7, the results from small trials may prove valuable in contributing to an overview of the evidence of treatment effectiveness, a view neatly summarized by Senn in the phrase 'some evidence is better than none'. Perhaps with clinical trials as with other things, size is not *always* everything.

3.6 Interim analysis

Many trials finish too soon, usually because the investigators run out of patients or money or both. But there are occasions when trials *should* finish before the intended completion date. Meinert (1986) makes the point that major ethical questions arise if investigators elect to continue a medical experiment beyond the point at which the evidence in favour of an effective treatment is unequivocal. Sadly however such situations do arise as is evidenced by the Tuskegee Syphilis Study. Initiated in the USA in 1932 and continued into the early 1970s, this study involved the enrolment and follow-up of 400 untreated latent syphilitic black males and 200 uninfected controls. The syphilitics remained untreated even after penicillin, an accepted effective treatment for the disease, became available. This was clearly indefensible, and led to the participants receiving a personal apology from President Clinton.

A clinical trial is, of course, a medical experiment, and it is ethically desirable to terminate such a trial earlier than originally planned if one therapy is clearly shown to be superior to the alternatives under test, or if a different concurrent study reports such a result. Patients assigned to the inferior treatment should be removed from it (and offered the superior treatment if appropriate) as soon as the evidence for a difference is clear. But as mentioned in the Introduction to this chapter, in most clinical trials patients are entered one at a time and their responses to treatment observed sequentially. Assessing these accumulating data for evidence of a treatment difference large and convincing enough to terminate the trial is rarely straightforward. Indeed the decision to stop accrual to a clinical trial early is often difficult and multifaceted. The procedure most widely adopted is a planned series of interim analyses of the data to be done at a limited number of protocol pre-specified time points during the course of the trial. Because the data are examined after groups of observations rather than after each observation, the name group sequential is often used for this procedure.

Interim analysis involves taking 'multiple looks' at accumulating data. The statistical problem is that of repeated tests of significance or multiple testing. The issue that arises is that, if on each 'look' the investigator follows conventional rules for interpreting the resulting P-value, the inappropriate rejection of the null hypothesis of no treatment difference will occur too often, that is there will be too many false positives. Or, as Cornfield (1976) has commented:

> Just as the Sphinx winks if you look at it too long, so, if you perform enough significance tests, you are sure to find significance even when none exists.

The problem of taking multiple looks at the accumulating data in a clinical trial has been addressed by many authors including Anscombe (1954), Armitage et al. (1969), McPherson (1983), Pocock (1983) and O'Brien and Fleming (1979). These authors point out that conventionally significant results (i.e. as judged by the usual threshold of say 5%) can often occur early on in a trial for a variety of reasons including:

- early patients in a trial are not always representative of the later patients;
- randomization may not yet have achieved balance.

An example of what can happen is provided by a trial designed to compare the efficacy of two antiretroviral agents (A and B) in HIV-infected patients described in Abrams et al. (1994). At the first interim analysis, carried out less than a year after the trial started, the results strongly favoured agent A; patients receiving it had experienced many fewer disease progressions and fewer deaths than those receiving the alternative. The nominal P-value associated with the treatment difference in progressions was an impressive 0.009. But after careful consideration the trial was continued and over time the differences favouring A steadily disappeared, so much so that at the end of the trial, the results had shifted from strongly favouring A to showing a small advantage for B.

The solution to the multiple testing problem associated with the ethical need for interim analyses in many clinical trials, is to define a critical value to be used at each planned interim analysis so that the overall Type I error rate is maintained at a prespecified level, for example, 0.05. The trial is continued if the magnitude of the test statistic is less than the appropriate critical value. The simplest approach would be to perform all interim tests at highly conservative levels (for example, require a P-value of 0.001 or less to justify early termination). Unfortunately this simple approach is too conservative to satisfy most investigators, and so several other sequences of critical values have been proposed, see, for example, Pocock (1977), O'Brien and Fleming (1979), Peto *et al.* (1976), Lan and DeMets (1983) and Pampallona and Tsiatis (1994).

Perhaps the most popular of these is that of O'Brien and Fleming, possibly because its properties reflect the thinking of experienced clinical trial investigators. Early interim analyses are very conservative requiring extremely low P-values to declare a significant result; this reflects the uncertainty and probable unreliability of any estimate of treatment early in the trial when the number of patients is small. As more patients are recruited the criteria for statistical significance become correspondingly less stringent and at the planned end of the trial (assuming it has not been terminated early) the critical value of the O'Brien-Fleming procedure is almost the same as would have been used in the trial if no interim analyses had been planned (Software is available for calculating the O'Brien-Fleming critical values and those for many of the alternative interim analysis procedures that are available—see Appendix C.).

The statistical guidelines governing the conduct of a series of planned interim analysis need to be clearly spelt out in the trial protocol. Unplanned interim analyses should be avoided at all costs as they can distort and discredit the results from even an otherwise well-designed clinical trial.

Interim analyses are designed to avoid continuing a trial beyond the point when the accumulated evidence indicates a clear treatment difference. As discussed above, this is clearly ethically desirable. But Pocock (1992) suggests that there is a real possibility that interim analyses claiming significant treatment differences will tend to exaggerate the true magnitude of the treatment effect and that often, subsequent analyses (where performed) are likely to show a reduction in both the significance and magnitude of these differences. His explanation of these phenomena is that interim analyses are often timed (either deliberately or unwittingly) to reflect a 'random high' in the treatment comparison. Simon (1994) also makes the point that estimates of treatment effects will often be biased in clinical trials that stop early.

Even though group sequential methods can be used to help decide when a trial should be stopped, the subsequent estimation of the treatment effect and its associated P-value still needs careful consideration. It is not difficult to find examples of trials in which some type of interim analysis was used to stop the trial early, but where the reported treatment effect estimate and its P-value were not adjusted for the sequential design but instead calculated as if the trial had been of fixed size (see, for example, Moertel *et al.*, 1990). Souhami (1994) suggests that stopping early because an effect is undoubtedly present may result in a serious loss of precision in estimation, and lead to imprecise claims of benefit or detriment. Methods that attempt to overcome such problems are described in Whitehead (1986), Rosner and Tsiatis (1989), Jennison and Turnbull (1989) and Pinheiro and DeMets (1997).

It was the Greenburg Report, finalized in 1967 but not published until 1988, that established the rationale for interim analyses of accumulating data. In addition, however, it emphasized the need for independent data monitoring committees to review interim data and take into consideration the multiple factors that are usually involved before early termination of a clinical trial can be justified. Such factors include baseline comparability, treatment compliance, outcome ascertainment, benefit to risk ratio, and public impact in addition to the results of an appropriate interim significance test. This type of committee is now regarded as an almost essential component of at least a sizable minority of clinical trials and helps ensure that interim analyses, by whatever method, do not become overly prescriptive (see Ellenberg et al., 2002).

The ethical need for planned interim analyses is most clear in trials that address major health concerns such as mortality, progression of a serious disease, or occurrence of a life-threatening event such as heart attack or stroke. Psychiatry trials with mortality as an endpoint are rare but such trials do occur. One example known to the authors involved a comparison of two drugs to treat patients with schizophrenia with the main question of interest involving the rate of sudden unexpected deaths with each treatment. Interim analyses using the O'Brien-Fleming approach and conducted when a pre-defined number of deaths had occurred, were part of the trial protocol.

The need for interim analyses is less convincing in many psychiatric trials that address symptom relief. And many experienced researchers working on trials in psychiatry might argue that the early declaration of an unequivocal treatment effect is unlikely since few trials in psychiatry have produced such a finding even on their completion! Nevertheless some examples of the use of interim analyses in a non-life threatening psychiatric context can be found; for example, in an investigation of the treatment of obsessive compulsive disorder, no significant difference between the two treatment groups on the Yale-Brown obsessive compulsive scale was found in a planned interim analysis, but the investigators considered that the trial should continue.

A slightly different aspect of the need to stop a trial early is raised by the question of unexpected adverse outcomes. In psychiatric trials this commonly involves the suicide of patients. Fortunately such events are rare in practice but they do occur, not least because nearly all psychiatric disorders are associated with an increased risk of suicide. Consequently it is inevitable that anyone who is actively involved in clinical trials in psychiatry will eventually have to confront the problem of a trial participant committing suicide. And it is almost as inevitable that shortly afterwards calls will be made for the trial to cease.

A practical example was encountered in one of the first trials of community versus hospital care for severe psychiatric illness that took place in the United

Kingdom, the Daily Living Programme Trial (DLP) (Muijen *et al.*, 1992). At that time stopping rules, Data Monitoring Committees (DMCs) and Trial Steering Committees (TSCs) were not as much part of the clinical trial scene as they are now. During the conduct of trial three participants committed suicide, and one committed a murder. This became national news, and there was much, frequently ill informed, newspaper coverage, linked with demands that the 'experiment' should cease forthwith. An internal inquiry was carried out by the hospital with the power to stop the trial but the trial continued, with some changes to the decision-making process relating to admission to the trial.

That decision to continue the trial seems justified even in hindsight. Suicides are rare events, and like many rare events follow what is known as a *Poisson distribution* (see Everitt, 2002*b*, for a definition and description), and apparent 'clusters' of events are often due to chance alone, rather similar to so-called 'cancer clusters' that also generate publicity and concern. There was no reason to think that the procedures of the trial added to the pre-existing risk. But what was learnt was the need to have clearer accountability and supervision. An independent oversight committee, established before it was needed, and involving major stakeholders including patient representatives, would almost certainly not have acted differently, but would have been better placed to provide reassurance to public, trial participants and investigators alike. Interim analyses of course would not have assisted, since the number of suicides and/or homicides that would have needed to occur to prove a causal link between the intervention and the adverse event would have been so high as to be almost inconceivable.

3.7 Summary

Designing a clinical trial requires considerable skill and attention to detail. Some of the issues that need to be dealt with have been covered in this chapter; a number of others particularly relevant to the design of trials in psychiatry will be addressed in Chapter 4. The details of the trial design and other aspects of trial management and so on, will need to be written up as the trial protocol, a topic that is taken up in Appendix A.

Chapter 4

Special problems of trials in psychiatry

4.1 Introduction

In the previous chapter, we looked in some detail at a variety of issues that are common to randomized controlled trials in whatever area they are used. In this chapter, we move from the general issues surrounding clinical trials to some more specific issues that are of particular concern to those undertaking trials in mental health.

Overall, the special problems of trials in psychiatry can be roughly divided into the simple and the complex, a division for which we are indebted to Mike Slade of the Institute of Psychiatry, London. The 'simple' problems are those that are amenable to technical solutions, even if in practice these can be hard to implement. For example, there is plenty of evidence of poor reporting of details of clinical trials performed in psychiatry (Gilbody *et al.*, 2002; Hotopf *et al.*, 1997). This would be rectified if more researchers followed the guidelines of the CONSORT statement (Altman *et al.*, 2001), as we have outlined elsewhere. Similarly, far too many trials in psychiatry are too short in duration. The simple solution, in theory at least, is to make them longer.

But there are also problems with psychiatry trials that are more fundamental. These include the necessary 'purity' of the RCT contrasted with the compromises and complexity of clinical care, and the arguments proposed by some that mental health interventions are so individual and personalized that they simply cannot be reduced to the generalizations necessary in an RCT. We will consider the latter arguments, which are essentially philosophical objections to the entire technology of trials, in our final chapter, but the former question, which is essentially one of generalizability, we will consider here.

Generalizability is indeed an important and thorny issue for mental health professionals; it involves the often difficult issue of the relationship between the world of trials and the world of clinical practice that the results of trials hope to inform. Confronting the issue requires a more detailed examination of the differences between pragmatic and explanatory trials, than was given when these terms were first introduced in Chapter 2.

4.2 Explanatory versus pragmatic trials

According to Roland and Torgerson (1998),

> Trials of healthcare interventions are often described as either explanatory or pragmatic. Explanatory trials generally measure efficacy—the benefits a treatment produces under ideal conditions, often using carefully defined subjects in a research clinic. Pragmatic trials measure effectiveness—the benefit the treatment produces in routine clinical practice.

In essence, an explanatory trial is designed to estimate the biological effect of a treatment, whereas a pragmatic trial is designed to estimate the effectiveness of a treatment in a target population. The eligibility criteria for an explanatory trial need to be chosen so as to minimize the impact of extraneous variation; consequently, such a trial needs to recruit as homogeneous a sample of participants as possible. The narrow eligibility criteria, often appropriate for an explanatory trial, can make it difficult (often impossible) to apply the results to a broader population.

In contrast, the participants selected for a pragmatic trial need to reflect variations between participants, that occur in real clinical practice, so that valid inferences can be drawn that are more likely to help to inform choices between treatments in a target population. A pragmatic trial does not attempt to add to understanding of disease or therapeutic mechanisms—it is instead intended to evaluate a simple question—'does this treatment work?' ignoring the supplementary question, 'and if so, how?' In particular, pragmatic trials are usually designed to reflect the realities of clinical practice, and to address one of the principal criticisms of many RCTs, namely their (perceived) lack of applicability to the 'real world' of clinical practice. Whilst this criticism is certainly not unique to psychiatry, it has perhaps been most often levelled against trials in the mental health context because of the frequently (and often strongly) expressed views that in this area in particular, most trials simply do not address clinical reality and so are not generalizable.

It is the issue of generalizability that is the principal driving force behind the call for more pragmatic trials in psychiatry and it is not difficult to find evidence why this is the case:

◆ Of all the manic patients admitted to one service, only 17% actually made it to the proposed clinical trial (Wentzer Licht et al., 1997). The patients randomized and those excluded differed on many characteristics. Those in the trial had less severe illnesses and less psychosis. Studies of patients entered into depression and schizophrenia trials have similar findings (Zimmerman et al., 2002; Woods et al., 2000). This is important, not because those in trials represent only a portion of the true population of those with psychiatric disorders—that is inevitable—but because the choice is not random, and is influenced by factors that relate to outcome.

◆ Patients excluded from community care trials are often those thought to be at high risk of suicide or homicide. Ironically, it is precisely in the treatment of such patients that clinicians need the most guidance (Taylor and Thornicroft, 2001).

♦ Outside the world of psychosis in the United Kingdom, the vast majority of people suffering from depression will be seen in primary care, and no other setting; those whose care is provided by specialist services are the exception, rather than the rule, and a selected and atypical exception at that. Yet, of the 13 829 trials listed on the trials register maintained by Cochrane Review Group for Depression, Anxiety and Neurosis, only 694 (5%) have a primary care setting.

The advent of modern diagnostic criteria poses additional problems. There is no doubt that introducing stricter diagnostic criteria into psychiatry has significantly aided research, especially into the causes of mental disorder. The late Robert Kendell was a fundamental influence in this respect. And, research is next to impossible unless one can be sure that like is being compared to like. But it can also have drawbacks. Psychiatrists have evolved a complex system of classification of depression, with categories such as dysthymia, melancholic depression, atypical depression, and so on. Yet in general practice, where the vast majority of depression is treated, it would be an exceptional doctor who was even aware of these subtleties, let alone using them. Instead, classification is generally pragmatic, using terms such as 'mild', 'moderate' or 'severe'.

Most trials however, as already described, take place in specialist settings, using the very same operational criteria that have little relevance to primary care. This is particularly so in the last decade. A recent review looked at the use of operational criteria in antidepressant trials. During the period from 1962 to 1970, no trials were reported that used such criteria; the corresponding figure for the 1990s was 94% (Barbui and Hotopf, 2001). In general, we salute the increasing precision of psychiatric diagnosis, but it poses a problem for studies that attempt to model real life clinical practice.

It is clear from the brief discussion above that clinical practice may differ from the conduct of randomized controlled trials in a number of ways, some of which we have identified, others of which are listed in Table 4.1 taken from Hotopf (2002).

Pragmatic trials exist to overcome at least some of these differences, by attempting to be as close to clinical reality as possible. The guiding principles are often simplicity and size, with the apotheosis of the pragmatic trial being the *large simple randomized trial* (see Chapter 8 and Hotopf *et al.*, 1999, for further discussion).

An example of how pragmatic trials work in practice is provided by the trial of treatments for depression in primary care reported in Ward *et al.*, 2000. The trial compared usual general practitioner care or up to 12 sessions of non-directive counselling or cognitive-behaviour therapy provided by therapists. As in all pragmatic trials, the researchers tried hard to make the participants as representative as possible of patients presenting with depression to primary care. Even so, only 464 of 627 patients presenting with depression, or with mixed anxiety and depression were suitable for inclusion (the main reason for exclusion being a score on the Beck Depression Inventory below the established cut off). It was also a patient preference trial, since, in real life, patients seen in primary care do express strong preferences for one form of treatment over another, even if there is no scientific evidence in favour of one or the other. The results were that 137 participants

Table 4.1 Some of the differences between routine clinical practice and traditional RCT design (reproduced with permission from Hotopf, 2002).

What happens in a typical RCT	What happens in the real world
Patients recruited from specialist centres, or by advertising	Patients are mainly treated in primary care
Patients with co-morbid medical or psychiatric disorders are excluded	Patients are probably treated, whatever comorbid disorders are there
Patients are carefully selected to generate homogenous diagnostic groups according to DSM or ICD	Patients with heterogeneous diagnoses according to DSM and ICD are 'lumped' together
Patients are allocated the treatment at random	Treatment is allocated via a complex process of explanation and negotiation
Patients are provided detailed information (which may be over-inclusive) for informed consent	Patients are provided brief information (which may be under-inclusive) for informed consent
Patients are given a one week 'placebo run in period' to remove placebo responders	All patients are given active treatment from the start
Placebo is used to compare active treatment	No placebo is used: choice is between active treatment and no treatment
Patients are followed at frequent intervals and given detailed check lists of side effects	Patients are followed at very varying lengths according to haphazard practice
Assessment endpoint is typically 4–6 weeks after treatment begins	Patient continued on treatment for 6 months, and the patient and the clinician are interested in much longer endpoints
Assessment of outcome is based on depressive symptoms and side effects	To the patient and the doctor, functional outcomes (e.g. return to work) may be more important
Patient and clinician are 'blind' to treatment group	Both (usually) are aware of the drug the patient is given

expressed clear preferences, and had to be allocated accordingly, 130 permitted a two-way randomization (not wishing to have usual care, but expressing no preference over counselling or CBT), leaving only 197 to agree to the full randomization. The conclusions from both the fully randomized and the patient preference arm were similar—an advantage to both psychological treatments over usual care at four months, but not at one year.

The protocols for both explanatory and pragmatic trials need to describe precisely the details of the intervention but in pragmatic trials this does not necessarily mean that the same treatment is offered to each patient. It may, for example, be the management protocol that is the subject of the investigation, not the individual treatments. For example, a recent trial studied the effects of giving general practitioners clinical practice guidelines on the risk of repetition of deliberate self-harm—there were none. (Bennewith *et al.*, 2002).

And it is not necessary (and sometimes not even desirable) for the patients to complete the trial in the group to which they were randomly allocated; it is however necessary that analysis involves the treatment groups as defined by randomization rather than by treatment eventually received, that is *intention to treat analysis* (see Chapter 5). Patients switching treatments may be an important marker for the limitations of the original treatment, but this information will be lost if they are analyzed in any way other than by initial allocation.

4.3 Complex interventions

The simpler the intervention, the easier the trial. The RCT methodology was developed principally for drug interventions, in which both intervention and control can be easily controlled and described. Later, the methodology was adapted for psychological interventions, the principal differences including the impossibility of ensuring double blindness, and the difficulties in ensuring treatment fidelity. Given that neither the therapist nor the patient can ever be blinded to the nature of a psychological treatment, an attempt has to be made to reduce observer bias by such stratagems, as using independent observers. Likewise, efforts are needed to ensure treatment fidelity, usually by use of manuals, taping sessions, and so on. But despite the best endeavours to match the operational simplicity of most drug trials, clinical trials that involve psychological therapies will almost always remain more complex than those involving drugs alone. And when we consider trials that test styles of healthcare delivery, as in models of community care, matters become even more problematic, so much so, that a literature has been developed around the nature and problems of what are now called 'complex interventions'.

What are complex interventions? The MRC provides a useful starting point (Anon, 2000):

> Health services have to evaluate a wide array of existing and newly proposed complex packages, so that the service can learn what is effective about any given intervention so that it can be more widely applied throughout the service. Some complex interventions are intended as improvements in the form of direct interventions at the level of individual patient care, for example a novel form of cognitive behavioural therapy. Other interventions, although ultimately intended to improve patient care, are actually delivered in the form of an organisation or service modification, for example the introduction of a physiotherapist or Parkinson's Disease nurse into primary care services. A third type of complex intervention is further removed again from individual patient care, although ultimately intended just as much to impact there, when an intervention is targeted on the health professional, for example, educational interventions in the form of treatment guidelines, protocols or decision aids.

Just as pharmacological trials have evolved their own jargon (see Chapter 2), so have complex interventions (Anon, 2000). And just as drug trials are now routinely described according to their place on the continuum from the earliest tests in human volunteers (Phase I studies) to post marketing surveillance (phase IV studies), developing and assessing complex interventions also passes through several stages:

♦ **Theory (or pre clinical).** Given that most evaluations of complex interventions in psychiatry are commenced after the intervention itself has been developed and/or implemented, occasionally as policy, the idea that one should develop the theoretical basis of the intervention as a first step is rarely, if ever, observed in practice. Sometimes, theory follows practice—What exactly are the active ingredients of CBT? What is the role of peer group influences in cessation of drug taking? Why do doctors fail to prescribe antidepressants at adequate doses?

♦ **Modelling.** This means developing an understanding of the intervention and its possible effects. Again, whilst in theory this can be paper or computer based, in reality it will involve small surveys, focus groups or observational studies.

♦ **Exploratory trial.** This is the most crucial stage, since many trials are often expensive, and are rarely undertaken without preliminary evidence from an exploratory trial in which evidence is collected on, for example, the appropriate control group, sample size calculations, outcome measures, and expected recruitment rates.

♦ **Definitive RCT.** This is much as it says, in which an appropriate RCT is designed fulfilling all the required standards of a well-designed trial.

♦ **Long-term implementation.**

The relationships between these categories are illustrated graphically in Figure 4.1.

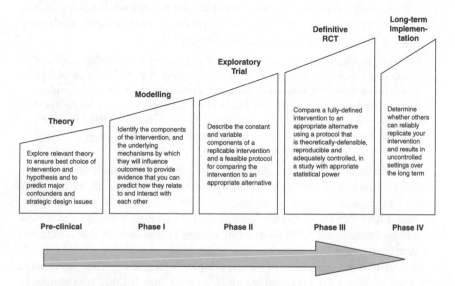

Fig. 4.1 A structural framework for development and evaluation of RCTs for complex interventions to improve health.

Clinical trials of complex interventions in psychiatry present several methodological challenges including deciding what were the active ingredients of therapy and why, ensuring the fidelity of the interventions, and managing variations amongst subgroups receiving the intervention (Crawford *et al.*, 2002). For example, we can be confident that if patients in a trial are randomized to, say, fluoxetine, then the characteristics of the medication will not differ between the recipients (assuming they take the medication). However, for complex interventions including the psychotherapies, this assumption is often not justified (Slade and Priebe, 2001), and may be next to impossible when the unit of analysis are services themselves (Slade *et al.*, 2002). Even when the intervention has been manualized, there can still be substantial differences between treatments given to patients under the same label (the issue of 'treatment fidelity'), and also, to put it simply, not all therapists are equally good.

Even after a study has taken place, there can be considerable debate about exactly what was being tested—as witnessed after the publications of two studies of different models of British community care—the UK-700 Trial and the PRISM study. In the former, some claimed that it was unclear whether or not this was an example of case management or assertive community care, whilst in the latter, a comparison of two different service configurations, there was considerable debate about what exactly was being tested.

4.4 Outcome measures in psychiatry

The outcome measure(s) used for treatment comparisons may be a clinical event, for example, death or recurrence of a disease, or a measurement of some characteristic of interest, for example, blood pressure, breathing difficulties, or depression. Such observations and measurements are the raw material of the trial, and they clearly need to be objective, precise, and reproducible for reasons nicely summarized by the following quotation from Fleiss (1986):

> The most elegant design of a clinical study will not overcome the damage caused by unreliable or imprecise measurement. The requirement that one's data be of high quality is at least as important a component of a proper study design as the requirement for randomisation, double blinding, controlling where necessary for prognostic factors and so on. Larger sample sizes than otherwise required, biased estimates, and even biased samples are some of the untoward consequences of unreliable measurements that can be demonstrated.

The problem of choosing appropriate and reliable outcome measures for use in clinical trials is not of course unique to mental health, but perhaps we in mental health have a particular skill of making things difficult for ourselves. Essentially, we have a tendency to try to measure too many outcomes, a tendency produced by mental illness being an inconveniently complex phenomenon that affects sufferers in many ways.

First, there is the experience of mental symptoms themselves. Then, there is the influence of illness on functioning, which in turn may include functioning in numerous domains – employment, home life, social life, and so on and so forth.

Mental illness is often a problem not only for the sufferer, but the rest of the family as well. These days, we also often ask about the costs of the intervention, and the sufferer's satisfaction with that intervention as well. Finally, time course adds extra dimensions of difficulty—psychiatric disorders remit and relapse, making measurement at a single time point unrealistically simplistic.

Each of these constructs is far from simple, and most have several dimensions. Few if any are 'all or nothing' phenomena, so beloved of trialists and statisticians. In a cardiology trial, assessing whether someone is dead or alive is easy, and can be done even if a person has been lost to follow-up. Statistically, death is a variable with only two data points, and lends itself to simple, clear statistical analysis (as Bradford Hill pointed out 'stone-dead has no fellow, and pre-eminent, therefore, stands the number of patients who die. No statistician, so far as I know, has in this respect accused the physician of an over-reliance on the clinical impression.'). Fortunately for the patients, death is not generally an issue in psychiatric trials. Instead, the variables measured in such trials are rarely simple, and are rarely measured in a simple fashion. Even what might appear to be a single outcome may in practice be more complex. A questionnaire measure of depression, or an assessment of family burden, for example, may consist of several different constructs.

The problem is that there are indeed many possible outcomes of mental illness. For example, a recent systematic review suggested that these could be divided into well being (Quality of life), cognition/emotion, behaviour, physical health, interpersonal, society, and services (Slade, 2002)—see Table 4.2.

If we want, for all the reasons that form a leitmotif of this book, to measure one pre defined outcome, which is it to be? And who should decide? There is a

Table 4.2 Health-related quality of life: what does it mean?

Concepts and domains	Definitions
HEALTH PERCEPTIONS	
Satisfaction with health	Physical, social and psychological function
General health perception	Self rating of health, health concern/anxiety
FUNCTIONAL STATUS	
Social	Work and daily role
Psychological	Distress (anxiety, depression)
Cognitive	Memory, reasoning, intellectual capacity
Physical	Activity restriction, fitness
MORBIDITY	
Signs observed	Objective clinical findings directly
Symptoms observable	Subjective evidence indirectly
Self reports conditions	Patient self report of symptoms and
Physiological diagnosis	Laboratory measures
DEATH AND DURATION OF LIFE	Survival

Source: Adapted from Gilbody, 2002; Patrick & Erickson, 1993.

modern trend to insist that these decisions should not, as in the past, be made by clinicians, but by patients themselves, and/or their carers. There is no fundamental objection to this, and much in favour, but will it lead to greater simplicity? Not necessarily—patients and carers are no more likely than clinicians to agree on a single outcome measure that encapsulates the complexities of mental disorders.

The consequence is that most, if not all, mental health trials use a package of measures, and will probably continue to do so. Many trials, for example, include some measures of symptomatic ill health, often linked to a diagnostic interview. There is usually an attempt to measure global functioning, an 'across the board' measure, which is often subdivided into various domains, such as social functioning or adjustment. These measures have some overlap with measures of quality of life, although the latter is designed to be particularly subjective—a snapshot of what the sufferer thinks about their illness, and their current life circumstances. In contrast, measures of functioning attempt to be more objective—looking at the effect of illness on various aspects of daily living and functioning. One or two have been designed specifically for single mental disorders—such as schizophrenia (Heinrichs et al., 1984) or depression (Hunt and McKenna, 1992).

It is also considered important to distinguish between psychiatric symptoms or psychopathology, and social functioning, which includes disabilities and handicap. One can have symptoms, but not be disabled. For example, studies of the outcome of adversity and disasters sometimes confuse the two—to be distressed after exposure to a disaster is exceptionally common, almost the norm, but to be disabled is not. The quintessential trauma-related psychiatric disorder, post traumatic stress disorder, requires the subject to be not solely symptomatic, but also disabled. Hence it is important that these two different domains are measured separately.

There are several texts nowadays which offer at least some guidance on the otherwise bewildering variety of outcome measures (Tansella and Thornicroft, 2001; Ishak and Burt, 2002; American Psychiatric Association, 2000; Farmer et al., 2002). However, we can make a general observation that the problem is not the lack of such measures, but the reverse. There are already too many scales available, and the number continues to rise. Over 640 have been used in schizophrenia trials (Gilbody et al., 2002). About a third of them were constructed specifically for the trial in question, and were not published at the time of being used. Intriguingly, those scales which had not been peer reviewed were significantly more likely to give statistically significant findings than those that had already been published in the literature (Marshall et al., 2000). And it is not surprising that as more scales become available, more are being used in individual studies. One study found that the mean number of outcome measures used in antidepressant trials has been rising by one per decade—a mean of one measure in the 1960s, rising to a mean of four in the last decade (Barbui and Hotopf, 2001).

We do not doubt that measuring outcome in psychiatry poses some problems. Nevertheless, a good motto is 'keep it short, keep it simple' (or alternatively, KISS, 'keep it simple, stupid'). Perhaps, psychiatry cannot go as far as the outcome scale for stroke studies devised by Charles Warlow, which uses three categories—'live and independent', 'live and dependent', and finally 'dead', but we could try. What patients, families, and clinicians want to know about treatment is not usually whether or not the new intervention causes a 20% reduction in base line score on the Positive and Negative Syndrome Scale (defined in most trials using this instrument as 'success'), but 'will this help me leave hospital, stay well, get a job or live independently from my family?' (Gilbody *et al.*, 2002). In general, psychiatrists appear to overestimate the importance of symptoms, possibly because of their key role in diagnosis, and underestimate the impact of psychiatric disorder on functioning and the ability to work (Kessler and Frank, 1997).

Outcome measures for trials therefore need to be made simpler. We cannot trace the origins of what has become the cliché of outcomes research—'the challenge is to make the important measurable, not the measurable important'[1] but even if it is cliché, it remains accurate. They need to reflect as closely as possible what clinicians, patients and families think are important, and to mirror those that are used in routine clinical practice and mental health settings (Richardson *et al.*, 2000; Slade, 2002). But even then, we anticipate that the problem of measuring too many outcomes will not go away.

Outcome measures are often best considered as divided into two classes:

♦ *Primary outcome measures*: the most important/relevant/practical that drives sample size calculations. This should be easy to measure or observe, free from ascertainment bias and clinically relevant.

♦ *Secondary outcome measures*: quality of life, safety, etc.

If we were finally able to solve the conundrum of measuring outcomes, would that remove the need for RCTs? Some have argued exactly that, saying that if only we could make all mental health services one large naturalistic experiment, with relevant outcomes data collected on every patient, there would be no need for RCTs at all (Ellwood, 1988). However, it should be crystal clear by now that we and others do not share that view (Dunn, 1996). Better measurement of outcomes, closer to those used in real clinical practice, will substantially improve the generalizability of clinical trials, but not the need for them in the first place.

4.4.1 Outcomes—objective or subjective?

The Holy Grail of outcomes research in psychiatry is to come up with a measure that is free from bias of any kind, reliable, easy to use, and adopted by trialists world wide. However, this nirvana has yet to be reached, and we are sceptical it ever will.

Take the most popular rating scale in mental health—the Hamilton Rating Scale for Depression (HRSD). It was developed some 40 years ago to evaluate the severity of illness in hospitalized patients (Hamilton, 1969). It is observer rated, and remains the gold standard outcome measure for clinical trials in depression, being used in nearly two thirds of modern depression trials (Snaith, 1996).

---

[1]It is sometimes ascribed to US Secretary of Defence Robert MacNamara during the Vietnam War, referring to the obsession with 'body counts', but we have been unable to verify this.

Yet, its popularity may owe more to habit and the fact that it has been used so often, than any inherent superiority over other measures. Because it was developed in hospital-based psychiatric practice in a different era, it is angled towards the more severe end of the spectrum of depressive disorders. A recent paper analyzed what would have happened if the criteria used in 39 antidepressant trials, taken from recent journals, had been applied to a non selective group of 1500 new psychiatric outpatients (Zimmerman *et al.*, 2002). The results showed that the two most common cut-offs used for the HRSD would have excluded almost half of the clinical sample, especially those towards the more moderate end of the spectrum. The authors also found that the proportion excluded varied from 11% to 71%, depending on the cut off used, illustrating another difficulty with the scale – the lack of consensus as to how it should be used. Another group of researchers identified 688 studies carried out between 1986 and 1992 that used the HRSD. Many employed modifications of the scale that have accrued over the years, with 11% of the studies failing to cite which modification they had used (Grundy *et al.*, 1994).

Another problem with the HSRD (and other observer rated scales in psychiatry) relates to the word 'objective'. It is easy to be persuaded that observer ratings are inherently more reliable than patient ratings, with the former being objective and the latter subjective. But things are not so straightforward. Depression is quintessentially a private, subjective experience. Using an observer does not per se add to objectivity. Instead, some have argued that it merely adds observer bias to all the other difficulties (Lewis, 1991) of observer rated scales, such as additional training for observers and measures to ensure inter rater reliability. Findings that the HRSD is 'more sensitive to change' than self-rated questionnaires may not necessarily mean that it is better, but could imply the opposite.

So the search for objective measures continues. A variety have been suggested—neuropsychological tests, electrophysiological measures, results from neuroimaging, and so on. In some, the proposed measure may have some validity—for example, the use of neuropsychological measures in trials of new treatments for dementia. But even here, trials have been criticized, and appropriately in our opinion, for over reliance on neuropsychological tests whilst disregarding outcome measures that really matter to patients and carers. We continue to be sceptical about the use of what are essentially proxy or surrogate measures for mental health outcomes, in which objective tests may lend some apparent objectivity and reliability, but often ignore feelings and behaviours, which are at the heart of mental disorders. Non-biological, patient-rated outcomes will remain the bedrock of clinical trials in mental health for sometime to come.

4.4.2 Outcome measure—when?

After an investigator planning a psychiatric trial has decided on the set of outcome measures to be made, there remains the crucial question of 'when' the measurements should be made. The timing of the measurement of outcome is a crucial one for psychiatry. In a cardiology trial of the immediate management of myocardial infarction, highly relevant and meaningful outcomes may be obtained within days, or certainly weeks. Unfortunately, there is a regrettable tendency in some psychiatric trials to follow the same model. Far too many trials in psychiatry report the effects of intervention on symptoms measured after only six weeks of therapy (why six weeks, we wonder?), whereas the natural history of psychiatric disorders tends towards chronicity, with conditions such as depression being comparable to disorders such as diabetes or rheumatoid arthritis in being potentially life long and requiring long-term management. Certainly, this is true for schizophrenia and the psychoses. Perhaps, psychiatrists should start to think about developing statistical measures that more accurately reflect the reality of chronic mental disorders that have alternating periods of good and poor functioning. A better way of appreciating this might be concepts such as areas under the curve, if the psychometric problems of multiple measurements could be overcome.

Likewise, too little attention is paid in psychiatric trials to the question of obtaining follow-up measurements that are adequate in number and duration. In our consulting work, we are often faced with clinicians bemoaning gaps in the outcome variables, sometime because when planning the trial they made no arrangements for ensuring adequate follow up, for example, such as obtaining consent for tracing.

4.5 Summary

At the start of the chapter we suggested that the problems with mental health trials come in two forms. Some are technical problems, which can be overcome with better education of trialists (uniform reporting standards), greater input from patients, and families (more relevant outcome measures) or more money (longer trials). Others require more thought about the purpose of RCTs in mental health. Are we testing whether or not a new intervention has the capacity to improve health—sometimes rather awkwardly called 'proof of principle'—or are we interested in whether or not the intervention really makes a difference to the lives of typical patients that mental health professionals try and help in real world settings? If we are interested in the latter—and to be frank, if we are not, then we should be—the answers lie in undertaking trials that are as close to real life clinical practice as possible (the pragmatic trial), and which deliberately embrace the complexity of mental health interventions (the science of complex interventions). Perhaps, more than any other branch of medicine, RCTs in mental health have to grapple with these difficult questions. However, we conclude the chapter by saying that although all of these are genuine difficulties to undertaking meaningful RCTs in mental health, none pose any insuperable objections to the fundamental principles of RCTs outlined so far. We shall return to some other general issues of psychiatric trials in Chapter 8.

Chapter 5

Some statistical issues in the analysis of psychiatric trials

5.1 Introduction

A clinical trial generates data that has to be analysed. Such analysis will involve the use of statistics, not always the most popular topic amongst clinicians and applied medical researchers, although few, we hope, would go as far as Le Fanu (1999) in believing that 'statistics are numbers to which complex mathematical formulae can be applied to produce conclusions of dubious veracity and from which all wit and human life is ingenuously excluded'. In this chapter we will examine a number of general statistical issues that we feel are of particular relevance in analysing data from psychiatric trials.

In essence, analysis and design are two sides of the same coin and if a poor design can make a clinical trial almost useless, the benefits of a good design can be undermined with a poorly planned (or executed) analysis. The practical implications of many of the points raised in this chapter will be illustrated in Chapter 6, where we describe in some detail the analysis of data from a specific psychiatric trial. (The material in the chapter is not intended as an introduction to the *technical* details of the statistical methodology used to analyse trial data; in fact we assume that readers will already have a reasonable grasp of many of the basic methods that might be used, for example, *t*-tests, regression etc. If they don't we recommend the texts on medical statistics by Altman, 1991, and Bland, 2000, and the more advanced and specific account of the statistics of trials given in Everitt and Pickles, 2000.)

5.2 *P*-values and confidence intervals

The *P*-value is probably the most ubiquitous statistical index found in the applied sciences literature and is, particularly, widely used in biomedical research. The *P*-value is defined as the probability of obtaining the observed data (or data that represent a more extreme departure from the null hypothesis) if the null hypothesis is true, and was first proposed as part of a quasi-formal method of inference by Fisher in his influential 1925 book, *Statistical Methods for Research Workers*. For Fisher the *P*-value represented an attempt to provide a measure of evidence against the null hypothesis; but Fisher intended it to be used informally with the smaller the *P*-value, the greater the evidence against the null hypothesis, rather than providing a division of the results into 'significant' and 'non-significant'.

Unfortunately it seems that despite the many caveats in the literature (see, for example, Gardner and Altman, 1986; Oakes, 1986), the accept/reject philosophy of hypothesis testing remains seductive to many clinicians (including psychiatrists), who seem determined to continue to express joy on achieving a *P*-value of 0.049, and despair on finding one of 'only' 0.051 (0.05 being the almost universally accepted threshold for labelling results, significant or non-significant). Many clinicians seem to internalize the difference between a *P*-value of 0.05 and one of 0.06 as 'right' versus 'wrong', 'creditable' versus 'embarrassing', 'success' versus 'failure' and, perhaps, the renewal of grants versus termination. Such practice was definitely *not* what Fisher had in mind as is evidenced by the following quotation in the 1925 edition of *Statistical Methods for Research Workers*:

> A man who 'rejects' a hypothesis provisionally, as a matter of habitual practice, when the significance is 1% or higher, will certainly be mistaken in not more than 1% of such decision . . . However, the calculation is absurdly academic, for in fact no scientific worker has a fixed level of significance at which from year to year, and in all circumstances, he rejects hypotheses; he rather gives his mind to each particular case in the light of his evidence and his ideas.

The most common alternative to presenting results from a clinical trial in terms of *P*-values, in relation to a statistical null hypothesis, is to estimate the magnitude of the difference of a measured outcome between treatment groups, along with some interval that includes the population value of the difference with some specified probability. Such an approach is intuitively sensible since most clinical objectives translate into a need to estimate a particular quantity, for example, a treatment effect, along with some idea of the precision of the estimate. The result is known, of course, as a *confidence interval*.

Confidence intervals can be found relatively simply for many quantities of interest (see Gardner and Altman, 1986), and although the underlying logic of interval estimation is essentially similar to that of significance testing, they do not carry with them the pseudoscientific hypothesis testing language of such tests. Instead they give a plausible range of values for the unknown difference. As Oakes (1986) rightly comments:

> the significance test relates to what the population parameter is not; the confidence interval gives a plausible range for what the parameter *is*.

According to Gardner and Altman (1986):

> Overemphasis on hypothesis testing—and the use of P-values to dichotomise significant or non-significant results—has distracted from more useful approaches to interpreting study results, such as estimation and confidence intervals. . . . The excessive

use of hypothesis testing at the expense of other ways of assessing results has reached such a degree that levels of significance are often quoted alone in the main text and abstracts of papers, with no mention of actual concentration, proportions etc., or their differences. The implications of hypothesis testing—that there can always be a simple 'yes' or 'no' answer as the fundamental result from a medical study—is clearly false, and used in this way hypothesis testing is of limited value.

Gardner and Altman's comments are well illustrated by the following quotation taken from a report of a clinical trial comparing olanzapine and haloperidol for treating the symptoms of schizophrenia:

> Patients treated with olanzapine showed an average decrease of 10.9 points on the Brief Psychiatric Rating Scale; patients treated with haloperidol reported an average decrease of 7.9 points. This difference was statistically significant.

Note neither a measure of the variation of the outcome measure is given nor an interval estimate of the treatment difference, i.e. a confidence interval.

Perhaps partly as a result of Gardner and Altman's paper, the use and reporting of confidence intervals have become more widespread in the medical literature in the past decade. Indeed many journals now demand such intervals rather than simply *P*-values. In many psychiatric journals, however, there appears to be a continuing commitment to *P*-values; certainly there is no discernable move away from their use. There should be.

5.3 Using baseline data

Pocock *et al.* (2002) point out that clinical trial investigators often record a great deal of baseline data on each patient at randomization. Such data can include, for example, details of previous disease events, current medication, age, sex, marital status, education etc. In addition it is very common to have one or more measurements of the main outcome variable(s) made before treatment begins. Baseline data collected in a clinical trial are often put to one (or more) of three possible uses:

• **Subgroup analysis**: here the aim is to explore whether there is any evidence that the difference between the treatments under investigation depends on any of the characteristics of patients included amongst the baseline data.

• **Covariate-adjusted analysis**: here the investigator attempts to take into account any of the baseline variables that are related to outcome in order to obtain a more precise estimate of the treatment effect. This analysis will be of most importance when a pre-randomization value(s) of the outcome measure is recorded, and in such cases it offers a far preferable analysis to the use of *change scores* as we shall indicate later.

• **Baseline comparisons**: a comparison of the baseline data in each treatment group usually to demonstrate that the treatment groups were similar prior to treatment getting underway.

Each of these uses of baseline data will now be examined more closely.

5.3.1 Subgroup analysis

The usual objective of a controlled clinical trial is to study the effects of a particular treatment given to patients of a particular type. The main conclusion from the trial is usually assumed to relate to any persons who meet the trial's eligibility criteria. But such a global statement may not be suited to the needs of individual patients and a question often posed is how to identify particular subgroups of patients for whom the optimal treatment differs from the overall patient population. For example, does a treatment work better for men than for women? Such a question is a natural one for clinicians since they do not treat 'average' patients and would, confronted with a female patient with a particular complaint, like to know, for example, whether the accepted treatment for the complaint works less well with women.

Testing whether the effect of treatment varies according to the value of one or more patient characteristics measured at baseline is relatively straightforward from a statistical point-of-view, but many statisticians would recommend that such analyses are best avoided altogether, or if undertaken, interpreted extremely cautiously in the sprit of 'exploration' rather than anything more formal (although the temptation to over interpret an apparent subgroup finding is likely to be difficult to resist—see Yusuf *et al.*, 1991). The reasons for their caution are not difficult to identify:

- Trials can rarely provide sufficient power to detect such sub-group/interaction effects; clinical trials accrue sufficient participants to provide adequate precision for estimating quantities of primary interest, usually overall treatment effects. Confining attention to subgroups almost always results in estimates of inadequate precision. A trial just large enough to evaluate an overall treatment effect reliably will almost inevitably lack precision for evaluating differential treatment effects between different population subgroups.

- Randomization ensures that the overall treatment groups in a clinical trial are likely to be comparable. Subgroups may not enjoy the same degree of balance in patient characteristics.

- There are often many possible prognostic factors in the baseline data, for example, age, gender, race, type, or stage of disease, from which to form subgroups, so that analyses may quickly degenerate into 'data dredging', from which arises the potential for *post hoc* emphasis on the subgroup analysis giving results of most interest to the investigator.

If subgroup analysis is undertaken it is important that appropriate tests of the treatment $\times$ covariate interactions of most interest are carried out appropriately. In particular, testing for a treatment difference separately in a number of subgroups (men and women again serve as a common example), and then comparing the resulting P-values is *not* valid. Each test assess the hypothesis of no treatment difference in a subgroup, but even when some of these are 'significant' and others are not, it does *not* imply that the treatment difference is *different* in each subgroup. The latter is only properly assessed by testing the significance of the appropriate treatment $\times$ covariate interaction. An example of sub-group analysis is given in Chapter 6. For further comments on the potential dangers of sub-group analysis see Pocock *et al.* (2002).

5.3.2 Covariate adjustment and change scores

Because randomization usually results in well balanced treatment groups, and experience shows that most potential covariates are not strongly related to the outcome, covariate adjustment in a clinical trial usually centres on what to do with the pre-randomization measures made on the outcome variable. These variables, except on very rare occasions, *will* be strongly related to outcome and it is important to use them correctly when analysing the data.

In the simplest situation a pre-treatment and post treatment value of the outcome measure are available for each participant in the trial. A popular procedure for dealing with such data, particularly it seems in psychiatry, is to base analyses on the *change score* (post minus pre, say). One of the arguments often used in favour of using change scores is that they deal with any imbalance between treatment groups in the baseline measurement. But the argument is false as is made clear by the following quotation from Senn (1997):

> Consider the case of a trial on blood pressure. If patients in one group in a trial of hypertension have a higher baseline measurement for systolic blood pressure on average than patients in another, then we should expect, other things being equal (including treatment effects) that they would also have a higher systolic blood pressure at trial outcome. We should not, of course, expect the difference between groups to be exactly the same at outcome as at baseline; although the correlation between the two is positive it is not, in general one.

It turns out, however, that because the correlation between baseline and outcome is generally less than one, the correlation between baseline and change score is generally negative. It then follows that an observed difference between groups at baseline is predictive not only of a difference in raw outcomes but also of a difference in change scores (albeit in the other direction). Hence, if the treatment is at an unfair disadvantage compared to placebo when its effects are measured in raw outcomes (due to an imbalance in baselines), it will have an unfair advantage if change scores are used.

The use of change scores corresponds to the assumption that the difference between the new treatment and standard treatment (or placebo) after treatment begins is, in the absence of a 'true' treatment effect, equal to the difference in the two treatments at baseline, prior to patients having received either treatment. In the context of many clinical trials, however, this assumption is likely to be false as is well documented by a number of authors, for example, Chuang-Stein and Tong (1997) and Senn (1994a, b). The reason is, of course, the *regression to the mean* phenomenon mentioned previously in Chapter 1. Here the term refers to the process that occurs as transient components of an initial score are dissipated over time. Selection of high scoring individuals for entry into a trial, necessarily also selects for individuals with high values of any transient component that might contribute to that score. Re-measurement during the trial will tend to show a declining mean value for such groups. Consequently, groups that initially differ through the existence of transient phenomena such as some forms of measurement error, will show a tendency to have converged on re-measurement.

Randomization ensures only that the treatment groups are similar in terms of expected values and so may actually differ not just in transient phenomena but also in more permanent components of the observed scores. Thus while the dissipation of transient components may bring about regression to the mean phenomena as previously described, the extent of the regression and the mean value to which the separate groups are regressing need not be expected to be the same.

Given these objections to the use of change scores, we might ask if baseline measurements can be used in *any* useful way in the analysis of clinical trial data, or should we deal simply with the post randomization values? The answer is, of course, that the baseline measurements *are* of value if they are used correctly. The approach to use is what is known as *analysis of covariance*. This type of analysis is described in detail in Altman (1991) and Senn (1997), but in essence it involves nothing more than fitting a relatively simple regression model with post treatment value as the dependent variable and as explanatory variables, pre-treatment score and treatment group represented by a dummy variable taking say the value 'one' for members of the active treatment group and 'zero' for those assigned to the alternative treatment or placebo group. Analysis of covariance has two distinct advantages over a simple analysis of change scores:

- It allows for a more general system of predicting what the post treatment difference would have been in the absence of any treatment effect as a function of the mean difference at baseline. Essentially the method produces a measure that is adjusted by baseline in such a way that the result is uncorrelated with baseline. Usually this corresponds to subtracting a fraction between zero and one of the baseline from the outcome measure.

- The analysis of covariance estimator has a variance that is generally lower than using simply the post treatment outcome or change scores; consequently analysis of covariance provides a more powerful analysis than either.

It is sometimes argued that clinical relevance may be used to decide between using change scores and analysis of covariance, or simply the analysis of the post randomization outcome. According to Senn (1998), 'this is just nonsense', since all these approaches measure the same thing, and for a trial, in which baseline values are perfectly balanced, give exactly the same answer. Furthermore, because it has the smaller variance, a covariance adjusted estimator from a given trial would actually be expected to predict the change score estimate in a subsequent trial, *better* than the change score estimator itself.

If the correlation (assumed the same in both treatment groups) between baseline measure of the response and the post treatment value is greater than 0.5, analysis of change scores remains less powerful than analysis of covariance, but is more powerful than analysing the post randomization measure only. If, however, the correlation is below 0.5, using change scores is *worse* than simply analysing the post randomization outcome alone. In such cases using change scores simply introduces more noise into the analysis. (The same arguments apply when there is more than a single pre-randomization baseline measure of outcome, and more than a single post randomization value recorded.)

Details of the mathematics behind these arguments, are given in Frison and Pocock, 1992, and Everitt and Pickles, 2000. In the latter some power curves are given showing the advantage of analysis of covariance over both analysis of change scores and analysis of the post treatment measures only, in terms of number of patients required to demonstrate a treatment effect of a particular size. Analysis of covariance requires fewer patients in all cases.

Despite the clear advantages of analysis of covariance for adjusting treatment effects for pre-treatment values of the outcome measure, Pocock *et al.* (2002) have found that many reports of clinical trials continue to analyse change scores, or simply ignore the pre-randomization outcome measures all together, a situation that needs to be corrected. (It should perhaps be noted that using the change score as dependent variable with the baseline as covariate in an analysis of covariance, gives exactly the same result as analysis of covariance using post randomization outcome with baseline as covariate—this analysis is often recommended by statisticians to clients who insist that they must work with change scores because of their clinical relevance!)

5.3.3 Baseline comparability

Many reports of clinical trials begin with a table in which baseline data are summarized by treatment group, often accompanied by a series of significance tests, one for each variable in the table. The reasons behind presenting such a table seem to include:

- To provide a description of the baseline characteristics of the sample of patients included in the trial.
- To demonstrate that randomization has worked well by achieving well balanced treatment groups at baseline.
- To identify any (unlucky) imbalances between treatment groups that may have arisen by chance.

The first of these bulleted points is entirely reasonable, since it is clearly important in assessing to whom the results of the trial can be applied, although it does not require the usual division of patient characteristics by treatment group, and certainly does not need the associated significance tests. The second and third points may also be largely sensible as long as any imbalances identified by examining the size of the *P*-values for each of the significance tests are *not* used to suggest possible covariates for adjusting the treatment effect. By definition, all baseline differences are due to chance (unless the randomization has gone wrong), and a statistical significant difference between treatment groups for a baseline variable is irrelevant when the baseline variable is not related to outcome. Conversely, imbalance for a strong predictor of outcome that is not statistically significant could matter.

Potentially important covariates should ideally be specified in the trial protocol, and chosen as a result of previous experience with the outcome measure to be used and its possible predictors. In practice, of course, this may not be so easy to arrange (see Pocock *et al.*, 2002). Certainly, however, covariates for adjusting the treatment effect in a clinical trial should *never* be chosen simply as a result of a small *P*-value when comparing the baseline data of the treatment groups. Indeed such *P*-values do not serve any useful purpose since they do not test a useful scientific hypothesis.

5.4 Longitudinal data

Medical treatments rarely result in a one time final result for a patient; generally they require clinicians to follow the evolution of a patient's health over a period of time. Consequently, in the majority of clinical trials the primary outcome variable(s) is measured on several occasions post-randomization and often also prior to randomization. Such *longitudinal studies* occupy a particularly important role in many areas of psychiatric research, not only clinical trials, but the methods used by psychiatrists to analyse such data are not always commensurate with the level of effort involved in their collection.

Longitudinal data arising from clinical trials can be (and have been) analysed in a variety of ways, some of which are more satisfactory than others, and in the last decade or so, many powerful new methods have evolved. It is important that psychiatrists involved in clinical trials become more aware of the possibilities such developments offer. In this section our aim is to give an informal, largely non-technical guide to what we see as the most suitable approaches to the analysis of longitudinal data, before, in Section 5.5, discussing particular problems arising in practice that complicate the picture. (We shall not cover obviously flawed methods such as 'time-by-time analysis' and 'end-point analysis', for reasons discussed by Everitt and Pickles, 2000, and by Gibbons *et al.*, 1993.)

5.4.1 Response feature analysis of longitudinal data

The *response feature* or *summary measure* approach to the analysis of longitudinal data is simple, straightforward and, in many cases, perfectly acceptable, particularly when only very few patients have missing values of the outcome measure, caused by either missing a scheduled visit or dropping out of the study altogether. (We will return to the missing value and dropout problem in Section 5.5.)

The essence of the summary measure method is to convert the repeated measurements of the outcome measure made post randomization, into a single measure that characterizes an important and relevant aspect of the participant's response. The chosen summary measure needs to be appropriate for the particular questions of interest in the trial and in the broader scientific context in which the study takes place. The key feature of a successful response feature analysis is the choice of a suitable summary measure, a choice that must be specified in the trial protocol before any data are collected.

A wide range of possible summary measures have been proposed; a number applicable to continuous outcomes are described in Table 5.1 (taken from Matthews *et al.*, 1990). Frison and Pocock (1992) argue that the *average* response to treatment over time is often likely to be the most relevant summary statistic in the majority of treatment trials.

Table 5.1 Possible summary measures (taken with permission of the BMJ Publishing Group from Matthews *et al.*, 1990, *British Medical Journal*).

Type of data	Question of interest	Summary measure
Peaked	Is overall value of outcome variable the same in different groups?	Overall mean (equal time intervals) or area under curve (unequal intervals)
Peaked	Is maximum (minimum) response different between groups?	Maximum (minimum) value
Peaked	Is time to maximum (minimum) response different between groups?	Time to maximum (minimum) response
Growth	Is rate of change of outcome different between groups?	Regression coefficient
Growth	Is eventual value of outcome different between groups?	Final value of outcome or difference between last and first values or percentage change between first and last values
Growth	Is response in one group delayed relative to the other?	Time to reach a particular value (e.g. a fixed percentage of baseline)

Having selected an appropriate summary measure, the analysis of the longitudinal data is thus reduced to a simple comparison of treatment group means on a single variable by way of a Student's *t*-test (two groups) or one-way analysis of variance (more than two groups). Pre-randomization measures, if available, can be incorporated into the analysis, by summarizing them in the same way as the post randomization measures, and then using an analysis of covariance on the pre- and post-randomization summary measures. An example is given in Chapter 6. (Further details of the summary measure approach are given in Everitt and Pickles, 2000.)

The statistical analysis of data from clinical trials should be no more complex than necessary. So in the case of longitudinal data, for example, the relatively straightforward summary measure approach described in this sub-section may not only be statistically and scientifically adequate for the estimation and testing of simple treatment differences, but will also often be more persuasive and easier to communicate to a general audience than more ambitious and sophisticated methods. It has to be recognized, however, that there may be occasions where the investigator wishes to pose more complex questions about the data collected in a longitudinal trial than can adequately answered by the response feature technique. More complex questions will require more complex methods of analysis to provide satisfactory answers, and in the next sub-section we describe one possibility.

5.4.2 Random effect models for longitudinal data

There are a number of desirable general features that methods used to analyse data, from studies in which the outcome variable is measured at several time points, should aim for including:

- The specification of the mean response profile over time needs to be sufficiently flexible to reflect both time trends within each treatment group and any differences in these time trends between treatments.

- Repeated measurements of the chosen outcome are likely to be correlated rather than independent and these correlations need to be properly accounted for to produce an analysis that is valid.

- The method of analysis should accommodate virtually arbitrary patterns of irregularly spaced time sequences within individuals (more will be said about this in Section 5.5).

There are a number of powerful methods for analysing longitudinal data that largely meet the requirements listed above. They all essentially consist of two components; the first component consists of a regression model for the average response over time and the effects of covariates such as treatment group, baseline measures, etc. on this average response, and the second component provides a model for the pattern of covariances or correlations between the repeated measures. Each component of the model involves a set of parameters that have to be estimated from the data. In most applications it is the parameters reflecting the effects of covariates on the average response that will be of most interest. But although the parameters modelling the covariance structure of the observations will not, in general, be of prime interest (they are often regarded as so-called *nuisance parameters*), specifying the wrong model for the covariance structure can affect the results that *are* of concern. Diggle (1988), for example, suggests that overparameterization of the covariance model component (i.e. using too many parameters for this part of the model) and too restrictive a specification (too few parameters to do justice to the actual covariance structure in the data) may both invalidate inferences about the mean response profiles when the assumed covariance structure does not hold. Consequently an investigator has to take seriously the need to investigate each of the two components of the chosen model.

Everitt and Pickles (2000) give full technical details of a variety of the models now available for the analysis of longitudinal data. Here we concentrate on just one approach, *the random effects model*, and try to make our account as low tech as possible!

Random effect models formalize the sensible idea that an individual's pattern of responses in a study is likely to depend on many characteristics of that individual, including some that are unobserved. These unobserved or unmeasured characteristics of the individuals in the study put them at varying predispositions for a positive or negative treatment response. The unobserved characteristics are then included in the model as random variables, i.e. random effects.

The essential feature of a random effects model for longitudinal data is that there is natural heterogeneity across individuals in their responses over time and that this heterogeneity can be represented by an appropriate probability distribution. Correlation among observations from the same individual arises from them sharing unobserved variables, for example, an increased propensity to the condition under investigation, or a predisposition to exaggerate symptoms perhaps. Conditional on the values of these random effects, the repeated measurements of the response variable are assumed to be independent, the so-called *local independence assumption*. (This assumption is not always valid and it is possible to build into random effect models a variety of residual error structures; see Pinheiro and Bates, 2001, for some examples.)

Such models become more transparent if we consider specific examples. Here we shall look at a simple situation in which, for a normally distributed outcome, we have observations over time for patients in two treatment groups. We wish to model the outcome at a particular time point, t_j, in terms of a simple linear regression on time, plus a covariate representing treatment group (this in the usual way will represented by a dummy variable taking values say 0 and 1, to label the two groups). To simplify the discussion we shall assume that there is not a group $\times$ time interaction. We shall examine two models, the *random intercept model* and the *random intercept and slope model*. (A little technical nomenclature will be used in describing the two models, but it is really little more than is generally used to describe the simple linear regression model-really!)

1 Random intercept model

Here the model for the response given by individual i at time t_j, y_{ij}, is modelled as:

$$y_{ij} = \beta_0 + \beta_1 \text{group}_i + \beta_2 t_j + u_i + \epsilon_{ij}, \qquad (5.1)$$

where group_i is the dummy variable indicating the group to which individual i belongs, β_0, β_1 and β_2 are the usual regression coefficients for the model; β_0 is the intercept, β_1 represents the treatment effect and β_2 the slope of the linear regression of outcome on time. The ϵ_{ij}s are the usual residual or 'error' terms, assumed to be normally distributed with mean zero and variance σ^2. The u_i terms are, in this case, random effects that model possible heterogeneity in the intercepts of the individuals, and are assumed normally distributed with zero mean and variance σ_u^2. (The ϵ_{ij} and u_i terms are assumed independent of one another.)

The model in eqn (5.1) is illustrated graphically in Fig. 5.1. Each individual's trend over time is parallel to their treatment group's average trend, but their intercepts differ. The repeated measurements of the outcome for an individual will vary about the individual's *own* regression line, rather than about the regression line for all individuals.

The presence of the u_i terms in eqn (5.1) implies that the repeated measurements of the response have a particular pattern for their covariance matrix; specifically the diagonal elements are each given by $\sigma^2 + \sigma_u^2$, and the off-diagonal elements are each equal to σ_u^2. The implication that each pair of repeated

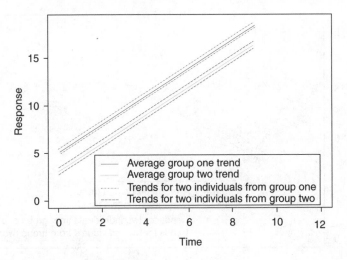

Fig. 5.1 The random intercept model.

measurements has the same correlation is not a realistic one for most longitudinal data sets. In practice it is more likely that observations made closer together in time will be more highly correlated than those taken further apart. Consequently for many such data sets the random intercept model will not do justice to the observed pattern of covariances between the repeated observations. A model that allows a more realistic structure for the covariances is one that allows heterogeneity in both slopes and intercepts.

2 Random intercept and slope model

In this case the model is given by

$$y_{ij} = \beta_0 + \beta_1 \text{group}_i + \beta_2 t_j + u_{i1} + u_{i2} t_j + \epsilon_{ij} \qquad (5.2)$$

Here the u_{i1} terms model heterogeneity in intercepts and the u_{i2} terms, heterogeneity in slopes. The two random effects are assumed to have a *bivariate normal distribution* with zero means for both variables, variances, $\sigma_{u_1}^2, \sigma_{u_2}^2$ and covariance $\sigma_{u_1 u_2}$. This model is illustrated in Fig. 5.2; individuals are allowed to deviate in terms of both slope and intercept from the average trend in their group.

This model allows a more complex pattern for the covariance matrix of the repeated measurements. In particular it allows variances and covariances to change over time, a pattern that occurs in many longitudinal data sets. (An explicit formula for the covariance matrix implied by this model is given in Everitt, 2002.)

Tests of fit of competing models are available that allow the most appropriate random effects model for the data to be selected—again see Everitt (2002) for details of such tests. In practice, however, changing the random effects to be included in a model often does not alter greatly the estimates of the regression coefficient (or coefficients) associated with the fixed effect(s) (β_1 in eqn 5.1 and 5.2)

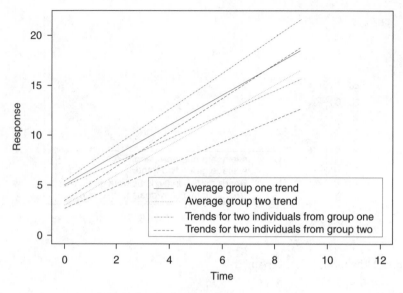

Fig. 5.2 The random intercept and slope model.

or their estimated standard errors. (Random effect models can also be used with non-normal response variables, in particular for repeated binary outcomes. The basis of analysis in this case is the usual *logistic regression model*. For details and examples see Everitt and Pickles, 2000, and Everitt, 2002.)

5.5 Missing values and dropouts in longitudinal data

In the majority of clinical trials in psychiatry involving longitudinal data there will be some patients who will miss one or more protocol scheduled visits after treatment has begun and so fail to have the required outcome measure made. There will be other patients who do not complete the intended follow-up for some reason and drop out of the study before the end date specified in the protocol. Both situations result in missing values of the outcome measure; in the first case these are intermittent, but dropping out of a study implies that once an observation at a particular time point is missing so are all the remaining planned observations. Many studies will contain missing values of both types, although in practice it is missing values that result from participants dropping out that cause most problems when coming to analysing the resulting data set. Missing observations are a nuisance when it comes to analysis and the very best way to avoid the problems they cause is not to have any! A few missing values caused by a small number of patients dropping out of a trial is unlikely to require much agonizing over how the resulting data should be dealt with, but when there are a substantial number of dropouts (not an infrequent occurrence in psychiatric trials—dropout rates in randomized trials of antidepressant drugs, for example, are often 30–40% over a three month course of treatment) careful consideration needs to be given to the implications that the resulting missing values have for analysis.

To understand the problems that patients dropping out can cause for the analysis of data from a longitudinal trial we need to consider a classification of dropout mechanisms based on the ideas in Rubin (1976). The type of mechanism involved has implications for which approaches to analysis are suitable and which are not. The classification involves three types of dropout mechanism:

- **Dropout completely at random (DCAR)**: here the probability that a patient drops out does not depend on either the observed or missing values of the response. Consequently the observed (non-missing) values effectively constitute a simple random sample of the values for all subjects. Possible examples include missing laboratory measurements because of a dropped test-tube (if it was not dropped because of the knowledge of any measurement), the accidental death of a participant in a study, or a participant moving to another area. Intermittent missing values in a longitudinal data set, whereby a patient misses a clinic visit for transitory reasons ('went shopping instead' or the like) can reasonably be assumed to be DCAR. Completely random dropout causes least problem for data analysis, but it is a strong assumption.

- **Dropout at random (DAR)**: The DAR mechanism occurs when the probability of dropping out depends on the outcome measures that have been observed in the past, but given this information is conditionally independent of all the future (unrecorded) values of the outcome variable following dropout. Here 'missingness' depends only on the observed data with the distribution of future values for a subject who drops out at a particular time being the same as the distribution of the future values of a subject who remains in at that time, if they have the same covariates and the same past history of outcome up to and including the specific time point. Murray and Findlay (1988) provide an example of this type of missing value from a study of hypertensive drugs in which the outcome measure was diastolic blood pressure. The protocol of the study specified that the participant was to be removed from the study when his/her blood pressure got too large. Here blood pressure at the time of dropout was observed before the participant dropped out, so although the dropout mechanism is not DCAR since it depends on the values of blood pressure, it *is* DAR, because dropout depends only on the observed part of the data. A further example of a DAR mechanism is provided by Heitjan (1997), and involves a study in which the response measure is body mass index (BMI). Suppose that the measure is missing because subjects who had high BMI values at earlier visits avoided being measured at later visits out of embarrassment, regardless of whether they had gained or lost weight in the intervening period. The missing values here are DAR but *not* DCAR; consequently methods applied to the data that assumed the latter might give misleading results (see later discussion).

- **Non-ignorable** (sometimes referred to as *informative*): The final type of dropout mechanism is one where the probability of dropping out depends on the unrecorded missing values—observations are likely to be missing when the outcome values that would have been observed had the patient not dropped out, are systematically higher or lower than usual (corresponding perhaps to their condition becoming worse or improving). A non-medical example is when individuals with lower income levels or very high incomes are less likely to provide their personal income in an interview. In a medical setting, possible examples are a participant dropping out of a longitudinal study when his/her blood pressure became too high and this value was not observed, or when their pain become intolerable and we did not record the associated pain value. For the BMI example introduced above, if subjects were more likely to avoid being measured if they had put on extra weight since the last visit, then the data are nonignorably missing. Dealing with data containing missing values that result from this type of dropout mechanism is difficult. The correct analyses for such data must estimate the dependence of the missingness probability on the missing values. Models and software that attempt this are available (see, for example, Diggle and Kenward, 1994) but their use is not routine and, in addition, it must be remembered that the associated parameter estimates can be unstable.

There are various possibilities when it comes to the analysis of longitudinal data where some of the patients dropout including:

- Discard incomplete cases and analyze the remainder—*complete case analysis.*

- *Impute* or fill in the missing values and then analyze the filled-in data.

- Analyze the incomplete data by a method that does not require a complete (rectangular) data set.

The first of these, complete case analysis, could not be simpler and was, at one time at least, a frequently used method for dealing with longitudinal data containing missing values. But complete case analysis is now no longer regarded by statisticians as respectable. The reasons are not difficult to identify. Complete case analysis only gives valid inferences when the dropout mechanism is DCAR, since then the complete cases are a random sub-sample of the original sample with respect to all variables. Even when the DCAR assumption is true however, complete case analysis remains objectionable. The rejection of the values of the outcome measure recorded, for people who eventually dropout, is an unnecessary waste of information that reduces the effective sample size, and makes any modeling and associated estimation process inefficient and sub-optimal. But such inefficiency of estimation may be a relatively minor cause for complaint against complete case analysis in comparison to the difficulties that arise when the dropout mechanism is *not* DCAR. In such cases (which are likely to be the majority), the complete cases are often a biased sample, with the size of the resulting bias depending on the degree of deviation from DCAR, the amount of missing data, and the specifics of the analysis.

Complete case analysis should now no longer be applied to longitudinal data with missing values; it is totally unnecessary since other more suitable alternatives are now readily available. The second approach to dealing with missing values caused by dropouts is imputation, a technique that is enthusiastically endorsed by Schafer (1999):

> Imputation, the practice of 'filling-in' missing data with plausible values, has long been recognized as an attractive approach to analysing incomplete data. . . . From an operational stand point, imputation solves the missing-data problem at the outset, enabling the analyst to proceed without further hindrance.

Certainly methods that impute missing values have the advantage that, unlike complete case analysis, observed values in the incomplete cases are retained. But some imputation methods can create more problems than they solve, possibly distorting parameter estimates, standard errors and hypothesis tests, so careful consideration is needed of which method to use. For example, a simple, and still commonly used method imputes missing values by the mean of the outcome for the values observed, perhaps calculated within a participant's own treatment group. But the only thing in favour of using this approach would be its simplicity. Even if the missing values arise from a DCAR mechanism (which is unlikely), this type of imputation will lead to say, confidence intervals and inferences which may be seriously distorted by bias and overstated precision (variances will clearly be underestimated, since the imputed cases contribute zero to the sum of squared deviations from sample means).

Another simple, and also widely used, imputation method is to replace the missing values due to a participant dropping out with that participant's last observed value. This is usually referred to as the *last observation carried forward* (LOCF) procedure. Clearly, this method makes a very strong assumption about the missing data, namely that the missing values on a case are all identical to the last observed value. Again this approach is likely to lead to a systematic underestimation of variability and is not recommended.

Neither the unconditional mean nor the LOCF imputation procedures should be used in practice for the reasons given above. More appropriate is some form of *multiple imputation*. This is a technique in which the missing values are replaced by more than one set of imputed values, usually between 3 and 10. In each case the missing values are predicted by applying some form of regression model extracted from the complete observations and adding in a random error component (full details are given in Schafer, 1999). Each of the 'complete' data sets is then analysed by standard methods and the results are later combined to produce estimates and confidence intervals that incorporate missing data uncertainty. In modern computing environments, the effort needed to produce and analyse a multiple-imputed data set is often not substantially greater than that required for single imputation. Suitable software is available—see Appendix C.

Complete-case analysis and imputation both result in a rectangular data matrix to analyze. At one time this was an important consideration since the methods (and software) used to deal with longitudinal data could only cope with situations in which each individual in the study had the same number of repeated measurements of the response, taken at the same time points. But this is no longer a requirement for current modeling techniques applicable to longitudinal data, in particular for the random effect models described earlier. Observations taken at a different set of time points for each subject can easily be accommodated and missing values can now be ignored in any analysis, without the *available* observations for an individual being excluded. (This is also true of the simple response feature approach described in Sub-Section 5.4.1.)

But under what type of dropout mechanism are the summary measure technique and random effect models valid when applied to longitudinal data with missing values? The former method requires the strong DCAR mechanism to hold to produce unbiased results, but the good news is that the latter approach can be shown to give valid results under the relatively weak assumption that the dropout mechanism is DAR (see Carpenter *et al.*, 2002).

When the missing values are thought to be informative, any analysis is potentially problematical but Diggle and Kenward (1994) have developed a modeling framework for longitudinal data with informative dropouts, in which random or completely random dropout mechanisms are also included as explicit models. The essential feature of the procedure is a logistic regression model for the probability of dropping out, in which the explanatory variables can include previous values of the response variable, and, in addition, the *unobserved* value at dropout as a *latent* variable (i.e. an unobserved variable). In other words, the dropout probability is allowed to depend on both the *observed* measurement history and the unobserved value at dropout. This allows both a formal assessment of the type of dropout mechanism in the data, and the estimation of effects of interest, for example, treatment effects under different assumption about the dropout mechanism. A full technical account of the model is given in Diggle and Kenward (1994) and a detailed example that uses the approach is described in Carpenter *et al.* (2002).

The Diggle-Kenward model represents a welcome addition to the methodology for analyzing longitudinal data in which there are dropouts. But as with any new methodology, questions need to be asked about its adequacy in practical situations. Matthews (1994), for example, makes the point that if there are many dropouts, the proposed model *can* still be applied, but questions whether many statisticians would feel happy to rely on technical virtuosity when say 60% of the data are absent. Alternatively, if the proportion of dropouts is low, then much less can be learnt about the dropout process, leading to low power to discriminate between dropout mechanisms. But despite these and other reservations that have been voiced about the Diggle-Kenward procedure, their proposed model does open up the possibility of some almost routine, detailed investigation of the dropout process and it will be used in the analysis of a particular psychiatric trial to be described in Chapter 6.

One of the problems for an investigator struggling to identify the dropout mechanism in a data set, is that there are no routine methods to help, although a number of largely ad hoc graphical procedures can be used as described in Diggle (1998), Everitt (2002*a*) and Carpenter *et al.* (2002). An example of the application of one of these graphical techniques will be given in Chapter 6.

5.6 Multiple outcome measures

The simplest randomized clinical trial involves the comparison of two treatments with respect to a *single* outcome measure. Unfortunately identifying a single primary outcome that adequately characterizes response to treatment may be difficult and, in many circumstances, an oversimplification of the diversity of patient response. In many disease conditions, response to treatment can have many different aspects. Consequently any associated clinical trials will lack a single definitive outcome measure that completely describes treatment efficacy. For example, O'Brien (1984) described a diabetes study in which 34 related response variables were considered necessary to characterize the treatment effect on nerve function. Certainly when a treatment is considered to affect a condition in a multitude of ways, several outcome variables may be necessary to fully describe its effects on patients. The multiple outcomes might include clinical events, symptoms, physiological measurements, blood tests, side effects, and quality of life. Pocock *et al.* (1987) found that over 30% of the 45 clinical trial reports they examined used more than six end points.

Most psychiatric trials will involve a variety of outcome measures, each possibly observed at several time points (see Chapter 4). Such multiple end points allow a more complete comparison of the merits of different treatments but increase the complexity of the statistical analyses required and can lead to problems of interpretation. Comparing treatment groups on each of the outcome measures separately, at some chosen significance level will inflate the type I error, i.e. the probability of rejecting the null hypothesis when it is true. For example, assuming that the measures are independent, testing five outcomes each at the 0.05 level will lead to an actual type I error of 0.226—the chance of a false positive finding is greatly increased. Various procedures have been proposed for keeping the probability that we reject one or more of the true null hypotheses in a set of comparisons (the *familywise error*, FEW) below of equal to a specified level α. The most familiar of these is the Bonferroni procedure which controls the FEW rate by conducting each test on an outcome measure at level α/m where m is the number of such measures. This procedure is very simple to apply but does have some drawbacks; the first of these is that it is excessively conservative, particularly of m is large. As a result there may be many tests significant at the a level but none at level α/m. In addition, the Bonferroni correction ignores the degree to which the outcome measures may be correlated; this again leads to conservatism when such correlations are substantial (see Blair *et al.*, 1996).

An alternative to testing each outcome measure separately at a significance level calculated to control the FEW rate, is to use a procedure that *simultaneously* tests for treatment differences on all outcomes. Such tests take into account the empirical correlation structure of the outcome measures, thus overcoming one of the criticisms of the Bonferroni procedure. The most well known of these global tests is *Hotelling's T^2*, the multivariate analogue of Student's *t*-test. The test is described in Everitt and Pickles (2000), but it is rarely used in clinical trials since it focuses on *any* departures from the null hypothesis, including those in which the directions of the differences might differ.

Pocock (1996) suggests that one possible approach to the multiple outcome problem would be pre-specification of priorities amongst the outcome measures. This would have the aim of providing a clear framework for emphasis (and deemphasis) of results in any eventual publication. Sadly, as Pocock points out, adhering to such priorities when results actually arrive might prove difficult for many. But organizers of trials should at least attempt to keep the number of outcome measures down to a reasonable number by clearly indicating the questions of greatest clinical interest. Awareness of the difficulties in both analyzing multiple outcomes and interpreting the results of such analysis should help to avoid an unnecessary excess of outcome measures being used. A report of a trial that includes a large number of significance test results generated by testing for a treatment difference on many, many outcomes does not generally make for convincing reading.

5.7 Intention-to-treat

In many clinical trials, not all patients adhere to the therapy to which they were randomly assigned. Instead they may receive the therapy assigned to another treatment group, or even a therapy different from any prescribed in the protocol. If such non-adherence occurs, care is required when assessing and estimating the treatment difference. There are a number of possible procedures that might be used, of which the following are the most common:

◆ *Intention-to-treat* or *analysis-as-randomized* in which analysis is based on original treatment assignment rather than treatment actually received. In detail intention-to-treat includes all randomized patients in the groups to which they were randomly assigned, regardless of their adherence with the entry criteria, regardless of the treatment they actually received, and regardless of subsequent withdrawal from treatment or deviation from the protocol. Intention-to-treat (ITT) analyses are therefore based on *allocated* treatment, rather than what treatment was actually given—it provides us with an estimate of the effect of offering treatment, as opposed to receiving it.

◆ *Adherers-only method*, i.e. analyzing only those patients who adhered to the original treatment assignment.

◆ *Treatment-received method*, i.e. analyzing patients according to the treatment ultimately received, even if randomization called for something else.

The intention-to-treat (ITT) approach requires that any comparison of the treatments is based upon comparison of the outcome results of all patients in the treatment groups to which they were randomly assigned. This approach is recommended by most statisticians and by regulatory authorities since it maintains the benefits of randomization. It also gives information relevant to the real world situation—if a large number of patients randomized to one arm of the trial either refuse or immediately drop out, then no matter how good the treatment was in those who chose to remain on it, in real clinical practice the treatment is unlikely to prove very successful.

In contrast, the second and third of the methods above compare groups that have *not* been randomized to their respective treatments; consequently, the analyses may be subject to unknown biases. But although it is clear that analyses based on compliance are inherently biased because non-compliance does not occur randomly, many clinicians (and even some statisticians) have criticized an analysis that does not reflect the treatment actually received, especially when many patients do not remain on the initially assigned therapy (see, for example, Feinstein, 1991). In the face of substantial non-compliance, it is not difficult to understand the intuitive appeal of comparing only those patients in the original trial that actually complied with the prescribed treatment. However, in addition to the difficulty of defining compliance in an objective manner, subjects who comply tend to fare differently and in a somewhat unpredictable way from those who do not comply. Thus any observed difference among treatment groups constructed in this way may be due not to treatment but to factors associated with compliance.

Dissatisfaction with analysis by original treatment assignment arises because of its apparent failure to evaluate the 'true' effect of the treatment. Some authors suggest that, an intention-to-treat analysis determines treatment effectiveness where this involves both compliance on treatment, as well as its biological effect, whereas an as-treated analysis assesses treatment efficacy. This, however, appears to simply be ignoring the potential problem of bias in the latter.

Peduzzi *et al.* (1993) compare the three methods of analysis described above on simulated data. One example presented involves simulated data for a hypothetical cohort of 350 medical and 350 surgical patients having exponentially distributed survival times and assuming a 10-year survival rate of 50% in each group. In addition, they generated an independent exponential time to 'crossover' for each of the 350 medical patients assuming half the patients crossed over by 10 years. Medical crossovers were then defined as those patients with time to crossover less than survival time. Fig. 5.3 displays 10-year survival rates by the as-randomized, adherers

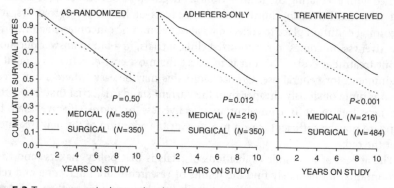

Fig. 5.3 Ten-year survival rates by the as-randomized, adherers-only, and treatment received approaches for a set of simulated data (taken with permission of John Wiley & Sons Ltd. from Peduzzi *et al.*, 1993, *Statistics in Medicine*).

only, and treatment-received methods. The latter two methods demonstrate a consistent survival advantage in favour of surgical therapy, when by definition here, there is actually no difference in survival between the two treatment groups.

According to Efron (1998), 'Statistics deals with the analysis of complicated noisy phenomena, never more so than in its applications to biomedical research, and in this noisy world the intent-to-treat analysis of a randomized double-blinded clinical trial stands as a flagpole of certainty amongst the chaos'. Indeed, according to Goetghebeur and Shapiro (1996), intention-to-treat analysis has achieved the status of a 'Buick'—'Best Unbiased Inference with regard to Causal Knowledge'. Many statisticians would endorse these views and also find themselves largely in agreement with Peduzzi *et al.* (1993):

> We conclude that the method of analysis should be consistent with the experimental design of a study. For randomized trials, such consistency requires the preservation of the random treatment assignment. Because methods that violate the principles of randomization are susceptible to bias, we are against their use.

It should be pointed out that intention-to-treat and the drop out problem in clinical trials are really best considered as separate issues. Intention-to-treat is synonymous with analysis as randomized, and could be applied both to data containing dropouts and data containing no dropouts. When applied to the former it does *not* require all the missing values to be imputed—say by LOCF, since the modelling techniques described earlier can all deal with data in which not all participants have measurements at the same set of time points. It is clear from reading trial reports in the psychiatric literature that many psychiatrists associate intention-to-treat with imputing data to get a rectangular data set, although the two are essentially *separate* issues to consider in the analysis of clinical trial data.

5.8   Economic evaluation of trials

At one time, researchers involved with clinical trials were almost exclusively concerned with evaluating the relative *clinical* effectiveness of competing treatments. But with the increasing burden on the budgets of health care providers, it is becoming common place to collect data about economic outcomes, in addition to effectiveness outcomes in randomized clinical trials, in a bid to answer questions about treatment costs. The aim is to select the most cost-effective treatment to recommend for general use. On occasions this may be easy; where a new treatment is quite obviously cheaper than the current standard, a trial that shows that the new treatment is equivalent in effectiveness or more effective than the standard may be sufficient reason to argue for the adoption of the new treatment over the old.

The appeal of economic evaluations of trials is that policy makers (and their accountants) immediately find the results of research more interesting and relevant, and may, as a consequence, be more likely to be persuaded by them. But both the measurement of cost and the evaluation of cost-effectiveness are far from straightforward.

5.8.1 Measuring costs

In practice routine audit systems rarely give adequate data for a proper evaluation of costs. Thus in practice, trials may need to include extended measurement protocols that can provide full treatment costs at the individual patient level. A variety of issues need to be borne in mind when considering these measures:

♦ Defining a cost is surprisingly complex. Are costs borne by patients rather than treatment providers to be included? Time off work might not be, but what about the costs of travel to receive treatment, or costs that are passed on directly from treatment provider to patient?

♦ Some costs are transfer costs and should not be included. Different treatments may involve a transfer in the billing of the same cost from one department to another, with no net change in cost.

♦ Costs should not be included for services that would not have been used elsewhere. For example, consider a new treatment that makes use of some currently rarely used but nonetheless necessary piece of equipment. Provided the use made of this equipment by the new treatment does not conflict with its current use, then much less than the full cost of this equipment should be attributed to the new treatment. The calculation of the appropriate amount, the so-called 'marginal opportunity cost', is often far from straightforward.

♦ Costs should not be counted twice. Thus drug costs charged to patients should not be included in both hospital costs and patient costs.

♦ In the same way that clinical outcomes are monitored and compared for a specified period of time, so too it is the case for costs. Longer term treatment benefits might include lower use, or sometimes greater use, of quite a range of health service facilities for complaints not obviously directly related to that treated. For example, patients with successfully treated heart conditions may experience longer term psychiatric problems that are costly to treat. Are these costs to be included? A further complication is that in most branches of economics it is usual to apply a discount rate to future costs, a reflection of the fact that where costs are deferred interest can be earned on the corresponding funds. What, if any, discount rate should be applied?

As a consequence of issues such as these, costs are easier to define within a small closed economic unit than within a community as a whole and can be substantially different. The cost of a treatment as viewed from the perspective of a single private health care provider can be very different from that viewed from the perspective of a national health service.

The uncertainties as to the inclusion criteria and amounts to assign makes this area of measurement one that should be subject to the same rigours as the rest of the trial protocol. This should include the need to define the range of eligible costs prior to randomization; the need for blindness in the collection of the economic data collection; and, particularly where the determination of unit costs is part of the analysis stage (i.e. are not known and agreed prior to the study), the importance of blindness and probably also 'independence' at the data-analysis stage.

5.8.2 Cost-effectiveness analysis

If measuring cost is difficult, no less so is the assessment of cost-effectiveness. Cost-effectiveness analysis attempts to measure the value of a new therapy by calculating the difference in cost between the new therapy and the standard therapy, divided by the difference in effectiveness of the two treatments (the *cost-effectiveness ratio*). Regression analysis is usually used to evaluate factors associated with cost. But the distribution of costs by patient is typically highly skewed, often with a small number of patients accounting for a disproportionate amount of the costs. For example, Fig. 5.4 shows the total costs (accommodation plus follow-up plus treatment costs) for the two treatment groups in a trial of cognitive-behavioural therapy (CBT) for pyschosis (Kuipers *et al.*, 1998). In both groups the costs distribution is skewed, but particularly so for the patients treated with CBT.

Some authors, for example, Hlatky *et al.* (2002), have recommended a log transformation of costs to deal with the skewness problem. However, others, including Everitt and Pickles (2000), have pointed out that economic cost has a scale that is fixed and known, with the consequence that analyses that attempt to deal with the non-normality of cost by transformation are not appropriate. The reason for this claim is that the estimated difference in log-costs of two treatments is not the same as the log of the estimated cost difference. The analysis of log costs simply does not answer the question of interest. Everitt and Pickles suggest that a better analysis of cost data in clinical trials is provided by using a generalized linear model approach and describe an example using data from the Kuipers *et al* (1998), CBT trial.

Another potential problem in analysing cost data from a clinical trial is that almost always, patient costs are derived by the application of unit costs to data on the number of units used by each patient. The units might include days and nights on an in-patient ward, number of outpatient assessments, units of blood products infused and so on. At least two potentially important consequences follow. Firstly, if there is variation in the costs of the same units between patients it is unlikely that this variation occurs at the patient level, but more often at the level of the medical centre, supplier or some such. Thus, from the point of view of costs, patients may

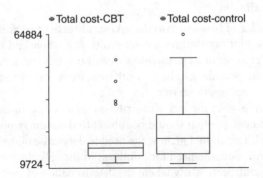

Fig. 5.4 Box-plots of the total cost for each treatment group in a clinical trial of cognitive behavioural therapy for psychosis.

fall within a much more complex sampling design, perhaps with nesting within centre, or within a crossed design of suppliers of different products or services. A failure to recognize such clustering may give a misleading impression as to the precision in the estimates of costs and cost differences. Secondly, and perhaps more importantly, there is typically considerable uncertainty in the costs of many of the units measured, and since the same unit costs are commonly applied across many or even all of the patients, a different choice of unit cost can substantially alter the overall results of a study. A common response to this problem is to narrow the focus of the analysis merely to those costs that can be well measured. Sometimes such costs represent a trivial proportion of the total costs and to narrow the focus in this way then makes very little sense. An alternative response is to consider a range of values for each unit cost, presenting the results in the form of a sensitivity analysis'. This typically provides results of little value, since it often results in few differences proving to be robust under the whole of the plausible unit cost space. One sensible way to approach this issue would be to formulate sensible distributions for unit costs and then to use these within a simulation based estimation method (see Everitt and Pickles, 2000, for details).

Rising health care costs have increased the pressure on physicians to consider the economic consequences of their medical decisions. Cost-effectiveness analysis is now an integral part of the assessment of treatments and addresses the question of whether a new treatment or other health care program offers good value for money. The development of statistical methods for the design and analysis of cost-effectiveness studies is a growth area and some recent examples include, Walker and Klassen (1995), Briggs *et al.* (1997), Briggs and Gray (1998), O'Hagan and Stevens (2002), Willian *et al.* (2002), Cooper *et al.* (2002), and O'Brien and Briggs (2002). More general discussion of the role of cost-effectiveness analysis in medicine is given in Russell *et al.* (1996).

All aspects of cost-effectiveness analysis from actually measuring costs, to choosing suitable and appropriate methods of analysis are problematical. The whole area of economic evaluation of treatments and cost-effectiveness analysis is developing rapidly and we have been able to give only a brief account of the field here. But psychiatrists considering undertaking a trial need to be aware that it is increasingly likely that treatment costs will need to be a part of their intended study.

When economic evaluation becomes of prime importance in a trial some authors, for example, Simon *et al.* (1995), have suggested that modifications of the orthodox randomized trial may improve its generalizability (see Chapter 2) and its relevance to policy decisions.

5.9 Summary

The analysis carried out on data collected from a clinical trial can range from the simple to the complex. Senn (1997), for example, points out that in its simplest form a clinical trial consists of a head to head comparison of a single treatment group and a control group to answer a well-defined question. The analysis of such a trial might then consist of applying a single significance test or constructing a single confidence interval for the treatment difference. In practice, of course, matters tend to be a little more complex and most clinical trials generate a large amount of data; recording multiple outcomes at several different time points, along with obtaining details of side effects, laboratory safety variables and demographic variables, quickly increases the likely complexity of the subsequent analyses. Consequently that there are a variety of statistical issues to be considered with when dealing with data from clinical trials in general and psychiatry in particular:

◆ *P*-values or confidence intervals? Confidence intervals are to be preferred although Johnson (1998) reports that only a tiny majority of clinical trial reports in psychiatry use them.

◆ Change scores or analysis of covariance? Analysis of covariance is more powerful and analysis of change scores cannot be defended.

◆ Which is the appropriate model for longitudinal data? Random effect models are one possibility and can be used to model the appropriate covariance structure for the repeated measures, thus allowing valid inferences to be made about the effect of treatment.

◆ What to do about dropouts? The dropout mechanism has implications for analysis, but identifying the mechanism is not always easy. And in many trials in psychiatry some patients may discontinue protocol treatment because of failure to improve or severe side effects, whilst others may improve rapidly and discontinue because of a perception that no further treatment is necessary. Consequently methods of analysis that make only relatively weak assumptions about the dropout mechanism, for example, random effect models, have a distinct advantage over those requiring stronger assumptions.

◆ Intention-to-treat or analysis by treatment received? Only intention to treat is acceptable. All patients randomized are included in the analysis according to their original assignment even if they have had their treatment changed shortly after randomization, or crossed over from one study treatment to another.

◆ How to estimate the cost effectiveness of a new treatment? Economic endpoints feature increasingly frequently in psychiatric trials, but they pose several methodological challenges, from how to measure cost sensibly to the most appropriate methods of analysis.

The practical implications of a number of the issues raised here will be illustrated in Chapter 6 by analysing in some detail, data from a particular psychiatric trial.

Chapter 6

Analysing data from a psychiatric trial: an example

6.1 Introduction

In Chapter 5, a variety of issues that might arise in the analysis of data from trials in general, and psychiatric trials in particular, were raised. In this chapter a number of these issues will be considered in the context of the analysis of data from a particular psychiatric trial described in Section 6.2. The main purpose of the analyses presented in this chapter is to illustrate the use of a variety of methods, including some that may not be familiar to all readers. In particular we will give special attention to the problems for analysis caused by patients dropping out of the trial, a problem introduced in Chapter 5. The analyses we describe here are not, of course, the only ones that might be applied to the data, and it might be a useful exercise for readers to apply other methods and then compare their results with ours.

6.2 Beating the blues

Readers of this book are unlikely to need to be reminded that depression is a major public health problem across the world. Antidepressants are the front line treatment, but many patients either do not respond to them, or do not like taking them. The main alternative is psychotherapy, and the modern 'talking treatments' such as *cognitive behavioural therapy* (CBT) have been shown to be as effective as drugs, and probably more so when it comes to relapse (Watkins and Williams, 1998). But there is a problem, namely availability—there are simply nothing like enough skilled therapists to meet the demand, and little prospect at all of this situation changing.

A number of alternative modes of delivery of CBT have been explored, including interactive systems making use of the new computer technologies. The principles of CBT lend themselves reasonably well to computerization, and, perhaps surprisingly, patients adapt well to this procedure, and do not seem to miss the physical presence of the therapist as much as one might expect. Workers at the

Institute of Psychiatry in the United Kingdom have developed one particular programme, known as 'Beating the Blues(BtB)'. Full details are given in Proudfoot *et al.* (2002), but in essence BtB is an interactive programme using multimedia techniques, in particular video vignettes. The computer based intervention consists of nine sessions, followed by eight therapy sessions, each lasting about 50 min. Nurses are used to explain how the programme works, but are instructed to spend no more than 5 min with each patient at the start of each session, and are there simply to assist with the technology. In a randomized controlled trial of the programme, patients with depression recruited in primary care were randomized to either the BtB programme, or to 'Treatment as Usual (TAU)'. Patients randomized to BtB also received pharmacology and/or general GP support and practical/social help, offered as part of treatment as usual, with the exception of any face-to-face counselling or psychological intervention. Patients allocated to TAU received whatever treatment their GP prescribed. The latter included, besides any medication, discussion of problems with GP, provision of practical/social help, referral to a counsellor, referral to a practice nurse, referral to mental health professionals (psychologist, psychiatrist, community psychiatric nurse, counsellor), or further physical examination.

A number of outcome measures were used in the trial, but here we concentrate on the *Beck Depression Inventory II* (BDI) (Beck *et al.*, 1996). Measurements on this variable were made on the following five occasions:

- prior to treatment;
- 2 months after treatment began;
- at 1, 3 and 6 months follow-up, i.e. at 3, 5 and 8 months after treatment.

The resulting data from 100 patients are shown in Table 6.1. (The data used in this chapter are a subset of the original and are used with the kind permission of the organizers of the study, in particular Dr Judy Proudfoot.)

The data in Table 6.1 have the following features that are fairly typical of those collected in many clinical trials in psychiatry:

- There are a considerable number of missing values caused by patients dropping out of the study.
- There are repeated measurements of the outcome taken on each patient post-treatment, along with a baseline pre-treatment measurement.
- The data is multicentre in that they have been collected from a number of different GP surgeries.
- The effect of the treatment in different subgroups is of interest-here, in particular, whether any treatment effect differs in patients where the duration of their current episode of depression was less than 6 months from those where it was greater than 6 months.

In the next section we will consider the analysis of only one of the post randomization measures of the BDI in Table 6.1, and then, in later sections, move on to deal with the full longitudinal complexity of the data.

89	< 6	BtheB	s4	33	13	13	10	8
90	< 6	BtheB	s6	19	4	27	1	2
91	< 6	TAU	s1	16	NA	NA	NA	NA
92	< 6	BtheB	s1	30	26	28	NA	NA
93	< 6	BtheB	s8	17	8	7	12	NA
94	> 6	BtheB	s1	19	4	3	3	3
95	> 6	BtheB	s1	16	11	4	2	3
96	> 6	BtheB	s5	16	16	10	10	8
97	< 6	TAU	s1	28	NA	NA	NA	NA
98	> 6	BtheB	s4	11	22	9	11	11
99	< 6	TAU	s4	13	5	5	0	6
100	< 6	TAU	s6	43	NA	NA	NA	NA

NA denotes a missing value

6.3 Analysis of the post-treatment BDI scores

Although few psychiatric clinical trials will involve the measurement of a single outcome on one occasion after treatment, we shall in this section consider only the post-treatment, two-month BDI score from the data in Table 6.1. This will allow us to remind readers of a few simple statistical procedures before moving on, in later sections, to consider increasingly complex and sophisticated analysis methods for the data.

Two sensible initial steps in investigating the outcome measure are:

♦ Calculate a number of summary statistics by treatment group—see Table 6.2.

♦ Construct some appropriate graphical displays of the data—two possibilities, histograms and box-plots, are shown in Figs 6.1 and 6.2.

The summary statistics and the graphical material both suggest that the average BDI score two months post-treatment is somewhat lower in the BtB group than in the TAU group. The score appears to have a moderate degree of skewness in both groups. Missing values are not a great problem for the 2 months post-treatment BDI score since only three patients have not had the score recorded, all of them in the TAU group.

Table 6.2 Summary statistics for BDI score at 2 months.

| | Treatment allocated | |
	BtB	TAU
Number of patients	52	48
Number of missing values	0	3
Mean	14.7	19.5
Median	12.5	20
Range	0, 40	0, 48
Standard deviation	10.1	11.1

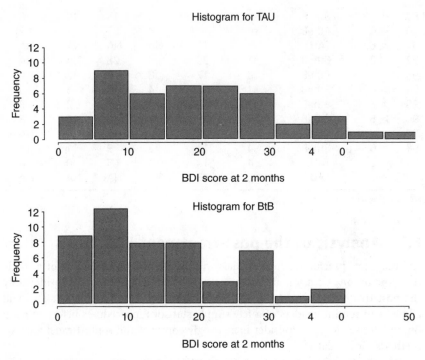

Fig. 6.1 Histograms of BDI scores at two months by treatment group.

Having made an initial informal examination of the data, the next step is to undertake a more formal investigation of how the two treatments differ in respect of the BDI score. This calls for the use of a statistical significance test, the calculation of the ubiquitous P-value, and/or the construction of a confidence interval for the treatment difference (our preference is for the latter for the reasons given

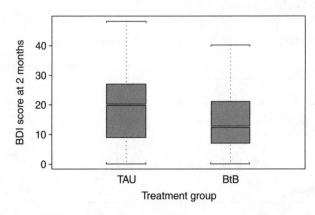

Fig. 6.2 Boxplots of BDI scores at two months by treatment group.

Table 6.3 *T*-test and confidence interval for difference in average BDI score in the two treatment groups.

Standard two-sample *t*-test

t	df	P-value
2.21	95	0.03

95% CI: (0.5, 9.0)

in Chapter 5, but since many readers may feel distressed unless they can look at the associated *P*-value, we will present both).

The most obvious test to use here is Student's independent samples *t*-test which will assess the null hypothesis that the population BDI means are the same for each treatment, BtB and TAU. The test is based on the assumptions of the normality of the BDI score in both the BtB and TAU treated populations and on its variance being the same in each population. It is this test that we shall use, despite the indication of a moderate departure from the assumption of normality suggested by the initial analyses of the data. Our justification for this apparent cavalier attitude to disregarding one of the assumptions of the *t*-test is the well-documented *robustness* of the test to a degree of non-normality of the observations.

The results of applying the *t*-test to the two-month BDI scores are shown in Table 6.3. There is evidence that the average BDI scores for the two treatment groups differ; the *P*-value associated with the *t*-test being 0.03. The corresponding confidence interval indicates that the average BDI score for patients treated with BtB is likely to be somewhere between 0.5 and 9 points lower than for those treated with TAU. So the existence of a 'statistically significant' difference between the groups is relatively clear. Of more interest and importance, however, is the *clinical* relevance of this difference, a point taken up later.

Now let us consider how we might extend the analysis of the BDI score at two months to include the measurement of BDI made before treatment began. A scatterplot of the two-month measurement against the pre-treatment value is shown in Fig. 6.3 and indicates, as might be expected, that they are relatively strongly related—patients with a high baseline depression value tend to have a high depression score at two months and vice-versa. Also shown on Fig. 6.3 are the estimated simple linear regression fits of BDI at two months on BDI pre for each treatment group—there is some suggestion that the two regression lines are not parallel.

One way many clinicians might incorporate the baseline BDI measurement into an analysis would be by the calculation of a *change score*, i.e. BDI at two months−BDI pre, for each patient. These change scores would then be used in place of the two-month BDI score in the analyses reported in Table 6.3. But for reasons described in Chapter 5 this is often a poor choice. A more powerful approach is to use the baseline BDI value as a covariate in an *analysis of covariance* of BDI at two months. This analysis is really nothing more than a linear regression of the two-month BDI score on two explanatory variables namely:

♦ BDI pre treatment,

♦ A dummy variable labelling treatment group—say 0 for TAU and 1 for BtB.

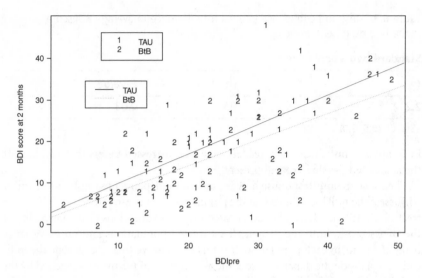

Fig. 6.3 Scatterplot of BDI score at two months against BDI pre-treatment, showing fitted linear regressions for each treatment group.

However, because of the evidence of non-parallel regression lines in Figure 6.3 we may also wish to consider the possibility of an *interaction* between treatment group and the baseline BDI score. An interaction in this context simply means that the effect of treatment is different for different levels of baseline depression.

The results from fitting regression models with and without a treatment × BDI pre-interaction are shown in Table 6.4. These results demonstrate that there is no convincing evidence of a treatment × pre-score interaction, so the observed divergence of the two regression lines in Figure 6.3 does not reflect a population

Table 6.4 Regression analysis for BDI at two months.

Covariate	Estimated regression coefficient	SE	t	P-value
(1) *BDI pre and treatment group*				
Intercept	3.10	2.03	1.53	0.13
BDI pre	0.60	0.08	7.60	< 0.001
Treatment	−3.95	1.71	−2.32	0.02
(2) *BDI pre, treatment group and interaction of baseline BDI with treatment*				
Intercept	2.55	2.10	1.22	0.23
BDI pre	0.62	0.08	7.59	< 0.001
Treatment	−0.20	4.20	−0.05	0.96
BDI pre × Treatment	−0.16	0.16	−0.98	0.33

Test of whether model two improves on model one has an associated P-value of 0.33, indicating that it does not.

difference. The result of regressing the two-month BDI score on the baseline value and the treatment dummy variable leads to the following estimated regression model:

Average BDI at two months = 3.10 + 0.60 BDI pre − 3.95 Treatment

The fitted model is shown in Figure 6.4. The estimated 95% confidence interval for the treatment effect, conditional on the equality of pre-treatment scores in the two groups is, −3.95 ± 1.96 × 1.71, i.e. (−7.30, −0.60). Treatment with BtB, lowers the average BDI score at two months by between about half a point to about seven points compared to TAU. The interval is quite similar to that calculated from the two months scores alone. A reduction of seven points in average BDI would be a clinically significant, and indeed a substantial improvement. On the other hand, if the 'true' reduction was only just over half a point, the use of the BtB programme may not be considered worthwhile, although this might depend on its cost-effectiveness. The clinician is left with the question 'the treatment appears to work, but does it work well enough?'

The full data set in Table 6.1 is *longitudinal* consisting as it does of a single pre-treatment value of the BDI for each patient, and 4 post-treatment values. We now move on to consideration of this aspect of the data, beginning in the next section with some useful graphical displays of the data, followed by the use of the summary measure approach described in Chapter 5. Then in Section 6.5 we fit some random effect models to the data. Finally, in Section 6.6 we confront the potentially tricky problem of the dropouts in the data.

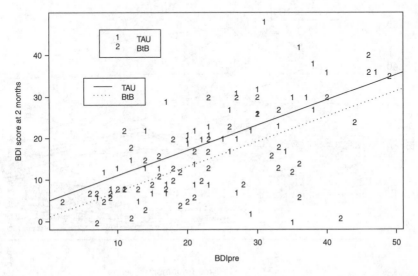

Fig. 6.4 BDI score at two months plotted against BDI pre-treatment, showing fitted model for the data.

6.4 Graphical displays and summary measure analysis of longitudinal data

Graphical displays of data are often useful for exposing patterns in the data, particularly when these are unexpected; this might be of great value in suggesting which class of models might be most sensibly applied in any later more formal analyses of the data. According to Diggle *et al.* (1994), there is no single prescription for making effective graphical displays of longitudinal data although the following guidelines are suggested:

- ◆ Show as much of the relevant raw data as possible rather than only data summaries.

- ◆ Highlight aggregate patterns of potential scientific interest.

- ◆ Identify both cross-sectional and longitudinal patterns.

- ◆ Make easy the identification of unusual individuals or unusual observations.

Here we give three graphical displays of the data in Table 6.1. The first in Fig. 6.5 shows the individual patient profiles over time. There is considerable variation between patients, even those in the same treatment group. The profiles demonstrate the phenomenon know as *tracking*; patients who were most depressed at the beginning of the study tend to be the most depressed throughout the study. There appears to be a steady decrease in the BDI scores over time in both treatment groups.

In Fig. 6.6 the group mean profiles and standard error bars for the data at each visit are shown. The gradual decline in the BDI over time is now very clear.

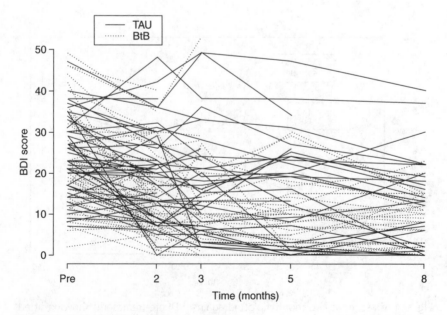

Fig. 6.5 Individual patient profiles for BtB data.

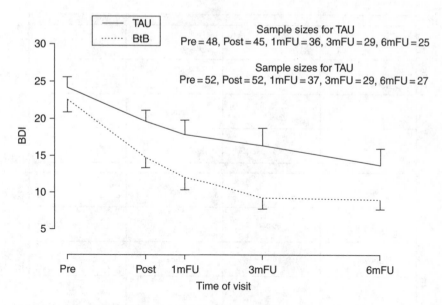

Fig. 6.6 Mean profiles for BtB and TAU treatment groups.

In addition it seems that the patients given BtB have a lower average BDI score at the 2 months post-treatment visit and that this difference is maintained and perhaps even increased over the three follow up visits.

Lastly in Figure 6.7 we show the *scatterplot matrix* of the 4 post-treatment BDI scores within each treatment group. Such a plot is often very useful in assessing the relationships between the repeated measurements and may give insights into their correlational structure that may prove helpful when it comes to fitting formal models to the data as we shall see in the next section. In this example, the pairs of repeated measurements are clearly strongly related with, apparently, a similar degree of correlation between each pair, a point we shall return to later.

The summary measure approach to analysing longitudinal data was introduced in Chapter 5. The essential feature of the method is to derive a single value from the repeated measurements available from each patient that captures some essential feature of the patient's response over time. In this way subsequent analyses are simplified. This approach has been in use for many years, and is described in Oldham (1962), Yates (1982), and Matthews *et al.* (1990). Various aspects of response feature analysis will be considered in this section including how to incorporate covariates, and the implication for the method of having missing values. But as mentioned in Chapter 5 the most important issue is the choice of a *suitable* summary measure, since this is usually the key to a successful analysis. The chosen summary measure needs to be relevant to the particular questions of interest in the study and in the broader scientific context in which the study takes place.

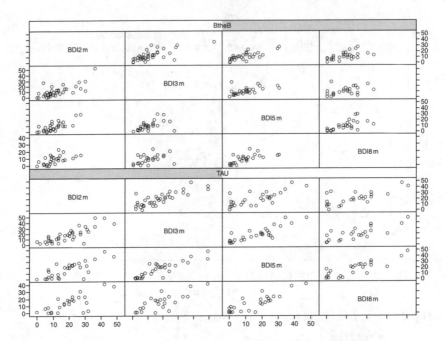

Fig. 6.7 Scatterplot matrix of post randomization BDI scores by treatment group.

In some longitudinal studies, more than a single summary measure might be deemed relevant or necessary, in which case the problem of combined inference may need to be addressed. More often in practice, however, it is likely that the different measures will deal with substantially different questions so that each will have a natural interpretation in its own right. (In most cases, the decision over what is a suitable measure should be made *before* the data are collected.)

A number of possible summary measures were listed in Table 5.1 in the previous chapter. Frison and Pocock (1992) argue that the average response to treatment over time is often likely to be the most relevant summary statistic in many treatment trials and it is this suggestion that we shall adopt here. Consequently the mean of the *available* post-treatment BDI scores for each patient will be calculated as our summary measure. These means are shown in Table 6.5. Note that the only missing values for our summary statistic correspond to the three patients for whom *none* of the intended 4 post-treatment BDI measurements were made. A boxplot of the means for the two treatment groups is shown in Fig. 6.8. There is some evidence of an outlier in the BtB group; this is patient 85 who has a value of 44.5. For the moment we shall retain this patient, and the results of applying a *t*-test to *all* available mean scores and the corresponding confidence interval for the treatment difference are shown in Table 6.6. The test is non-significant and the confidence interval includes the value zero. The implication is that there is no treatment difference, although the lower limit of the confidence interval being just below zero and the upper limit nearly eight points above zero, might be

Table 6.5 Means of available post-treatment BDI values for each patient.

Subject	Treatment	Mean of available post-treatment BDI scores
1	TAU	2.00
2	BtB	19.25
3	TAU	20.00
4	BtB	13.00
5	BtB	23.00
6	BtB	6.00
7	TAU	18.25
8	TAU	14.50
9	BtB	7.50
10	BtB	17.50
11	TAU	35.00
12	BtB	25.00
13	TAU	27.75
14	TAU	15.25
15	BtB	4.50
16	TAU	29.50
17	BtB	7.25
18	BtB	29.00
19	TAU	10.00
20	BtB	6.00
21	BtB	16.50
22	TAU	16.00
23	TAU	21.00
24	TAU	23.00
25	TAU	12.50
26	BtB	15.00
27	TAU	39.66
28	TAU	2.00
29	BtB	5.00
30	BtB	9.50
31	TAU	8.500
32	BtB	7.00
33	BtB	7.00
34	BtB	21.75
35	BtB	38.00
36	TAU	10.75
37	TAU	11.75
38	TAU	4.00
39	BtB	24.00
40	TAU	40.00
41	BtB	18.50
42	TAU	7.75
43	TAU	20.00
44	BtB	6.25

Table 6.5 (continued)

Subject	Treatment	Mean of available post-treatment BDI scores
45	BtB	30.00
46	BtB	22.00
47	BtB	0.33
48	BtB	5.00
49	BtB	44.50
50	TAU	30.00
51	TAU	20.00
52	BtB	40.25
53	TAU	6.00
54	BtB	23.50
55	TAU	4.00
56	BtB	13.50
57	TAU	34.50
58	TAU	30.00
59	BtB	3.00
60	BtB	19.00
61	TAU	20.00
62	TAU	11.00
63	TAU	16.33
64	TAU	18.00
65	BtB	3.00
66	TAU	3.25
67	TAU	17.00
68	BtB	20.00
69	TAU	30.00
70	BtB	4.25
71	BtB	21.00
72	BtB	7.50
73	TAU	8.00
74	TAU	21.50
75	TAU	15.00
76	BtB	11.50
77	BtB	8.00
78	BtB	9.00
79	TAU	22.75
80	TAU	23.75
81	TAU	15.00
82	BtB	13.25
83	TAU	5.75
84	TAU	44.50
85	BtB	12.75
86	BtB	17.00
87	BtB	1.75
88	TAU	11.00

89	BtB	8.50
90	BtB	NA
91	TAU	27.00
92	BtB	9.00
93	BtB	3.25
94	BtB	5.00
95	BtB	11.00
96	BtB	NA
97	TAU	13.25
98	BtB	4.00
99	TAU	NA
100	TAU	2.00

Table 6.6 Results of t-test, confidence interval and analysis of covariance for means in Table 6.5.

1. Standard two-sample t-test

t	df	P-value
1.65	95	0.10

95% confidence interval, $(-0.73, 7.84)$

2. Analysis of covariance

Covariates	Estimated regression coefficient	Standard Error	t value	P-value
(Intercept)	1.24	1.97	0.63	0.53
BDIpre	0.63	0.08	8.22	< 0.001
Treatment	−2.72	1.66	−1.64	0.11

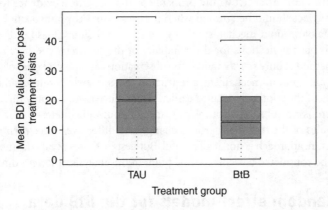

Fig. 6.8 Boxplots of post-treatment mean values for the patients in each treatment group.

Table 6.7 Results of *t*-test, confidence interval and analysis of covariance for means in Table 6.5 after removal of patient 85.

1. Standard two-sample *t*-test

t	df	*P*-value
1.99	94	0.05

95% confidence interval, (0.016, 8.29)

2. Analysis of covariance

Covariates	Estimated regression coefficient	Standard error	*t* value	*P*-value
(Intercept)	1.89	1.97	0.96	0.34
BDIpre	0.60	0.08	8.69	< 0.001
Treatment	−3.08	1.64	−1.88	0.06

suggestive of a 'tendency' for patients on TAU to have higher post-treatment BDI scores than those on BtB.

The baseline BDI value can be incorporated into the summary measure approach using the same type of regression model as was used in the previous section. This result is also shown in Table 5.7. The confidence interval for the treatment difference, conditional on equality on average baseline score is now (−0.54, 5.97). Again there is no real evidence of a treatment effect.

Repeating the analyses shown in Table 6.6 after removing patient number 85 gives the results shown in Table 6.7. The *t*-test is now just significant at the 5% level and associated confidence interval has a lower limit marginally greater than zero. This analysis produces some relatively weak evidence of a treatment effect. But the new analysis of covariance again suggests that there is no treatment difference. The clinical verdict would probably be that statistical evidence for a small treatment effect should be ignored when it arises from dropping a single patient.

The type of dropout mechanism that gives rise to missing values (as discussed in Chapter 5) has implications for the suitability of the summary measure approach, and the method is only *strictly* valid if the observations are missing due to a dropout completely at random mechanism, a restriction that somewhat counters the attractive features of the approach detailed earlier. (Here, since there are only three missing values there is no substantial problem.) And, of course, if interest lies in how the mean profiles of the treatment groups change and differ over time, then the summary measure approach is not at all helpful. But despite these caveats the method can still often be considered a useful starting point in the analysis of longitudinal data.

6.5 Random effect models for the BtB data

It cannot be overemphasized that statistical analyses of clinical trials should be no more complex than necessary. So even when longitudinal data have been collected, it is not always essential to apply an analysis that deals explicitly with the repeated measures aspect of the data. For example, there are often occasions when the summary measure approach used in the previous section provides a perfectly adequate analysis. Nonetheless, a typical trial does not take place in a scientific vacuum in which a simple treatment difference is the only question of interest. It is more usual that, in addition to being used as the basis of formal evidence for efficacy or equivalence, even a phase III trial will gather data that may be informative as to the mode of action of the treatment, dose–response relationship, response heterogeneity, side effects, and so on. In addition, attrition and variation in compliance may need to be more carefully examined than can be done within, for example, the simple summary statistic approach.

In this section we shall describe the application of a variety of random effect models to the BtB data. (These models were introduced in Chapter 5.) A small rearrangement of the data puts them into a form that makes it more transparent how the models to be applied operate. The rearranged data for the first five patients in Table 6.1 is shown in Table 6.8. The data in Table 6.8 is said to be in the 'long' form.

Before considering random effect models for the data, we will fit a multiple regression model that simply ignores the fact that patients have repeated measures of the BDI, i.e. it assumes that the BDI measurements are independent. With the data reorganized into the long form, such an analysis is extremely

Table 6.8 Data from first five patients in Table 6.1 in 'long' form.

	Subject	New surg	New treatment	New drug	New length (months)	Newpre	Visit	BDI
1	1	s1	TAU	No	> 6	29	2	2
2	1	s1	TAU	No	> 6	29	3	2
3	1	s1	TAU	No	> 6	29	5	NA
4	1	s1	TAU	No	> 6	29	8	NA
5	2	s2	BtheB	Yes	> 6	32	2	16
6	2	s2	BtheB	Yes	> 6	32	3	24
7	2	s2	BtheB	Yes	> 6	32	5	17
8	2	s2	BtheB	Yes	> 6	32	8	20
9	3	s3	TAU	Yes	< 6	25	2	20
10	3	s3	TAU	Yes	< 6	25	3	NA
11	3	s3	TAU	Yes	< 6	25	5	NA
12	3	s3	TAU	Yes	< 6	25	8	NA
13	4	s4	BtheB	No	> 6	21	2	17
14	4	s4	BtheB	No	> 6	21	3	16
15	4	s4	BtheB	No	> 6	21	5	10
16	4	s4	BtheB	No	> 6	21	8	9
17	5	s4	BtheB	Yes	> 6	26	2	23
18	5	s4	BtheB	Yes	> 6	26	3	NA
19	5	s4	BtheB	Yes	> 6	26	5	NA
20	5	s4	BtheB	Yes	> 6	26	8	NA

Table 6.9 Results of fitting a model that assumes post-treatment measures of BDI are independent.

Covariate	Estimated regression coefficient	Standard error	t value	P-value
(Intercept)	5.54	1.62	3.41	0.001
BDIpre	0.55	0.05	10.79	< 0.001
Visit	−0.94	0.24	−3.90	< 0.001
Treatment	−4.58	1.06	−4.31	< 0.000

simple to carry out using any of the major statistical software packages. Note that in this analysis all the observations that a patient actually has are retained, unlike what happens in the flawed complete case analysis approach described in Chapter 5.

The results from fitting a simple multiple regression model for BDI score, using BDI pre, visit (with values 2, 3, 5 and 8 months) and treatment (0 = TAU, 1 = BtB) as explanatory variables are shown in Table 6.9. We shall not spend time interpreting these results since they have been derived under the unrealistic assumption that the repeated measurements of the BDI variable are independent. The correlation matrix of these measurements shown in Table 6.10, and the scatterplots given previously in Figure 6.7, show that this is clearly not the case.

A more realistic model for the data is the random intercept model described in Chapter 5. The results of fitting a series of such models are shown in Table 6.11. It appears that a model involving only the main effects of baseline BDI, time and treatment is needed to describe the data adequately. Interaction terms such as time × treatment and BDI pre × treatment are not needed in the model.

The random intercept model implies a particular structure for the covariance matrix of the repeated measures, i.e. variances at the different visits are equal, and covariances between each pair of visits are equal. In addition the covariance matrix is assumed to be the same in both treatment groups. In general these are rather restrictive and unrealistic assumptions—for example, covariances between observations made closer together in time are likely to be higher than those made at greater time intervals. Consequently we might try a random intercept and slope model (as described in Chapter 5) to see if it describes the data better. The results are as shown in Table 6.12. For these data such a model does *not* provide an improvement in fit over the simpler random intercept model. Examining the

Table 6.10 Correlation matrix of repeated measures.

	BDI2m	BDI3m	BDI5m	BDI8m
BDI2m	1.00	0.74	0.79	0.70
BDI3m	0.74	1.00	0.82	0.72
BDI5m	0.79	0.82	1.00	0.81
BDI8m	0.70	0.72	0.81	1.00

Table 6.11 Results for a series of random intercept models fitted to the BtB data.

Covariate	Estimated regression coefficient	Standard error	t value	P-value
Model 1[a]				
(Intercept)	3.89	2.01	1.94	0.05
BDIpre	0.62	0.08	8.14	< 0.0001
Visit	−0.71	0.15	−4.79	< 0.0001
Treatment	−3.23	1.62	−2.00	0.05
Model 2[b]				
(Intercept)	3.90	2.02	1.93	0.06
BDIpre	0.62	0.08	8.09	< 0.0001
Visit	−0.71	0.15	−4.87	< 0.0001
Treatment	−5.02	1.94	−2.58	0.01
Visit × treatment	0.50	0.29	1.70	0.09
Model 3[c]				
(Intercept)	3.39	2.06	1.64	0.10
BDIpre	0.64	0.08	8.17	< 0.0001
Treatment	0.48	1.98	0.12	0.90
Visit	−0.71	0.15	−4.79	< 0.001
BDIpre × Treatment	−0.16	0.15	−1.02	0.31

[a] $\hat{\sigma}_u = 7.13$, $\hat{\sigma} = 5.01$
[b] $\hat{\sigma}_u = 7.21$, $\hat{\sigma} = 4.95$
Test of model 1 versus model 2: P-value = 0.09—model 2 does not significantly improve the fit
[c] $\hat{\sigma}_u = 7.07$, $\hat{\sigma} = 5.01$
Test of model 1 versus model 3: P-value = 0.30—model 3 does not significantly improve the fit

covariance matrix of the repeated measures—see Table 6.13—we see why. In this case it appears that the variances and covariances of the repeated measurements *do* approximate the structure required by the random intercept model, a fact already suggested by the scatterplot matrix in Figure 6.7.

Table 6.12 Results from a random intercept and slope model fitted to the BtB data.

Covariate	Estimated regression coefficient	Standard error	t value	P-value
Intercept	3.89	2.01	1.93	0.05
BDIpre	0.62	0.08	8.13	< 0.001
Visit	−0.71	0.15	−4.57	< 0.001
Treatment	−3.266	1.62	−2.02	0.05

$\hat{\sigma}_{u_1} = 7.33$, $\hat{\sigma}_{u_2} = 0.42$, $\hat{\sigma} = 4.89$: estimated correlation of u_1 and u_2 is −0.22
Test of model 1 in Table 6.12 versus this model: P-value = 0.81—this model provides no improvement in fit over model 1

Table 6.13 Covariance matrix of post-treatment BDI measures.

	BDI2m	BDI3m	BDI5m	BDI8m
BDI2m	105.70	79.35	88.77	67.33
BDI3m	79.35	108.21	93.78	69.89
BDI5m	88.77	93.78	120.80	82.92
BDI8m	67.33	69.89	82.92	86.59

Note that for both random effect models, the standard error of the treatment effect approaches *double* the corresponding value for the independence model as given in Table 6.8. This is intuitively what might be expected since the correlations between the repeated measurements lower the effective sample size compared to the same number of independent observations.

Up to now we have conveniently ignored the fact that data in the BtB study were collected from a number of different general practice surgeries, i.e. it is essentially a multicentre trial (see Chapter 3). We now need to consider the possibility that because of the possible different intake of patients etc. that results, particularly the treatment effect may differ between surgeries. Differences between surgeries and possible surgery × treatment interaction, *could* be investigated by taking surgery as a factor with eight levels and including it in the regression analysis, suitably coded, as a series of dummy variables. But suppose that instead of the eight surgeries there had been 30 or 50? In such cases using surgery as a factor with the 30 or 40 levels coded as dummy variables would provide a very poor analysis (consider, for example, how many variables would be involved in the regression model). A far better method is to model possible surgery differences and surgery × treatment interaction using random effects. For those readers who can bear a little algebra the two models we shall consider can be written as follows:

1. Surgery effect

$$y_{ijk} = \beta_0 + u_{1i} + u_{2k} + \beta_1 \text{ Treatment}_i + (\beta_2 + u_{3i}) \text{ time}_j + \epsilon_{ijk}, \quad (6.1)$$

2. Surgery × Treatment interaction

$$y_{ijk} = \beta_0 + u_{1i} + u_{2k} + (\beta_1 + u_{4k}) \text{ Treatment}_i + (\beta_2 + u_{3i}) \text{ time}_j + \epsilon_{ijk} \quad (6.2)$$

where y_{ijk} represents an observation of BDI made on subject i at time j in surgery k, and the u's represent the various random effects. In particular, in the first model, u_{2k} represents the surgery random effect that will cause patients within a surgery to be more similar to each other in respect of BDI values, than to patients in other surgeries. And in the second model, u_{4k} × treatment allows for the possibility of treatment effects being different in different surgeries.

In the first of these two models, the surgery random effect models possible level differences in BDI in different surgeries; these might arise when some surgeries are in deprived areas where there were generally higher depression levels, whereas others have a less depressed cliental. The second model introduces a further random effect term that models possible different treatment effects in the different surgeries. The latter would represent a treatment × surgery interaction that, if substantial, would perhaps give some cause for concern since it could imply that the treatment worked in some surgeries but not in others.

Fortunately for the data in Table 6.1, fitting the models specified in eqn (6.1) and (6.2) showed that surgery effects were not needed. Consequently the final model chosen to describe the average profiles of BDI scores in the two groups over the 4 post-treatment visits is as follows:

Average BDI at a particular visit $= 3.89 + 0.62$ pre $- 0.71$ visit $- 3.23$ treatment

This provides a concise, quantitative description of what is going on in the data:

◆ Conditional on treatment and visit, BDI *increases* on average by 0.62 (95% CI, [0.47, 0.76]) for each increase of one in the BDI pre score.

◆ Conditional on treatment and pre BDI, BDI after treatment *decreases* on average by 0.71 (95% CI, [0.42, 1.00]) for each increase of a month in time post-treatment.

◆ Conditional on visit and BDI pre, BDI is lower by an average of 3.23 (95% CI, [0.06, 6.40]) for patients treated with BtB compared to TAU.

In particular, treatment with BtB decreases BDI score by somewhere between a fraction over zero and just over six units on average, a difference that is the same at each post-treatment visit since there is no evidence of a treatment × visit interaction.

The analyses described above have essentially been concerned with answering the overall question as to whether the BtB program can, on average, decrease depression amongst the type of patient recruited into the trial. But clinicians looking at the data may raise other questions, for example, does the new treatment work better on those patients who have had their current episode of depression for less than six months? A subgroup analysis might be requested, despite the known weaknesses of such an approach (see Chapter 5). As an illustration of the possibilities some further random effect models, now including a dummy variable for duration of current episode (<6 m, >6 m) and the interaction of this variable and treatment, were fitted to the BtB data. The results are shown in Table 6.14. The treatment × length of current episode interaction term fails to reach

Table 6.14 Random intercept models including duration of episode and interaction of treatment with duration of episode.

Covariate	Estimated regression coefficient	Standard error	t value	P-value
Intercept	3.83	2.01	1.90	0.06
BDIpre	0.61	0.08	8.04	< 0.001
Visit	−0.71	0.15	−4.82	< 0.001
Treatment	−2.98	1.60	−1.86	0.07
Duration	0.80	1.64	0.49	0.63
Duration × Treatment	−2.76	1.60	−1.73	0.09

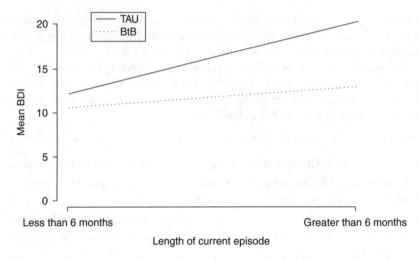

Fig. 6.9 Interaction plot of treatment means for BDI for patients with different lengths of current episode.

significance at the 5% level, although it is close enough to perhaps warrant a little 'data dredging' to look at a plot of treatment means for patients having a current episode of less than six months compared to those for which length of current episode is greater than six months. This plot is shown in Fig. 6.9. There appears to be some suggestion that the BtB program works better for those patients who have a longer duration current episode.

6.6 The dropout problem in the BtB data

In the BtB data in Table 6.1 there are a total of 47 patients who dropout of the study, 23 from the TAU group and 24 from the BtB group. What are the implications of these dropouts for the analyses reported in the previous section? Recall from Chapter 5 that for the random effect models to give valid results the dropout mechanism has to be DAR (or, of course, the weaker, DCAR). Carpenter *et al.* (2002) consider a number of tabular and graphical methods for assessing dropout mechanisms. One very simple graphical procedure will be illustrated here. The method involves plotting the observations for each treatment group, at each time point, differentiating between two categories of patient; those who do and those who do not attend their next scheduled visit. Any clear difference between these two categories in the plot would indicate that dropout is not completely at random. For the BtB data the resulting plot is shown in Fig. 6.10. There appears to be no very clear distinction in the distribution of BDI values of those patients who do and those who do not attend their next schedules visit. There is certainly no evidence in the plot of those who dropout at a particular time point having consistently higher (or lower) BDI values at the previous time point than those patients who are observed at *both* time points. The pattern in Fig. 6.10 is consistent

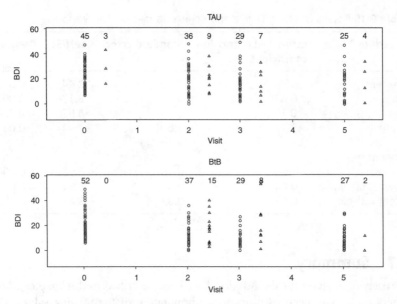

Fig. 6.10 Beat the blues data by treatment group and time, identifying patients who do (o) and do not attend (△) their next scheduled visit.

with a dropout completely at random mechanism given some reason for encouragement that the results from fitting the random effect models are valid.

The dropout mechanism can be investigated more formally using the approach popularized in Biostatistics by Diggle and Kenward (1994) and mentioned briefly in Chapter 5. (This approach has become more accessible with the development of suitable software such as GLLAMM as described in Rabe-Hesketh *et al.*, 2002; details are given in Appendix C.) With this approach, a logistic regression model is used for the probability of dropping out at a particular time point. A *latent variable* is included in the model to allow the probability of dropping out to depend on the unobserved value of the response at time of dropout. (The details of how this is possible are mathematically complex, but essentially involve an assumed distribution for the latent variable and then integration over this distribution.) Finding that the probability of dropping out depends on the latent variable would indicate an informative dropout mechanism (see Chapter 5) and throw the results from fitting the random effect models given earlier into doubt.

Fitting the Diggle-Kenward model to the BtB data leads to the results shown in Table 6.15. Here there is no evidence that the probability of dropping out depends on the latent variable, but there is evidence that this probability *does* depend on the previous value of BDI. Hence this more formal analysis suggests that the dropout mechanism is DAR, rather than DCAR as indicated by the earlier graphical method. Fortunately the random effect models only require the DAR assumption for their results to be valid. The estimated regression parameters for treatment, visit and pre BDI remain largely the same as in the analysis described previously.

Table 6.15 Results of fitting Diggle and Kenward's method for dropouts.

Covariate	Estimated regression coefficient	Standard error	Coeff/SE	P-value
Intercept	5.36	2.20	2.44	0.015
BDI pre	0.61	0.07	8.19	< 0.0001
Visit	−0.75	0.15	−4.97	< 0.0001
Treatment	−3.11	1.60	−1.94	0.052
Dropout model				
Intercept	−1.28	0.16	−8.02	< 0.0001
Previous BDI value	0.04	0.01	3.64	< 0.001
Latent variable	−0.02	0.02	−1.41	0.159

6.7 Summary

A variety of analyses for the BtB data have been described in this chapter. Many others could have been used, including imputation of the missing values. The methods of analysis used in this chapter may not all be familiar to psychiatrists undertaking clinical trials, particularly perhaps the use of random effect models for longitudinal data. (A further example of the use of the technique in psychiatry is given in Sensky *et al.*, 2000.) But such methods can now be used routinely because of the wide availability of suitable statistical software and they offer a very powerful approach to the analysis of longitudinal data. For such data, dropouts are frequently a problem and it is important that some attempt is made to investigate the likely dropout mechanism. Random effect models assume only that this mechanism is DAR rather than requiring the stronger DCAR assumption. Exploration of the dropout mechanism can be made by informal, usually graphical methods (see Diggle, 1998; Carpenter *et al.*, 2002), and by formally fitting the Diggle-Kenward model. Although this exploration requires some effort on the part of the investigator, it should be undertaken more often than it is in psychiatric trials that generate longitudinal data. After all, clinicians would not think of limiting themselves to the medical methods and techniques that were available 50 years ago, so why should they ignore recent relevant developments in statistical methodology in favour of *t*-tests, chi-square tests etc., that pre-date even Fisher's agricultural experiments?

Chapter 7

Systematic reviews and meta-analysis

7.1 Introduction

By now we hope all readers will agree on the need for methodological rigour if one is to establish if treatment A works better than treatment B for a particular condition using a randomized clinical trial. We hope also that most will agree that any such trial should conform to certain standards, and that those standards should be clearly expressed and reproducible. Opinions that 'something worked', or that 'we thought overall the patients improved/liked the intervention/didn't develop too many side effects' and so on are unacceptable because they are liable to bias.

But consider the situation when we are dealing not with a single trial, but with a review of many trials. Given that it is rare indeed that any single trial ever gives the definitive answer to a clinical question, it is via reviews of several trials that we finally arrive at a conclusion about the effectiveness or not of an intervention.

So we might reasonably expect that reviews, which after all are far more widely read by practising clinicians, who rarely have the time or the expertise to evaluate and synthesize each individual trial, should be as, and perhaps more, rigorous, than the individual trials that they involve. Sadly, until relatively recently, this expectation was rarely met.

In a pivotal paper Mulrow (1987) showed that looking only at four of the best medical journals, 86% of review articles depended upon qualitative synthesis of the literature, and only a handful contained any description of the methodology or rules by which papers were selected and conclusions reached. Since then numerous studies have showed again and again the deficiencies of the single, 'narrative review'. There is evidence that such narrative reviews can sometimes tell us more about the background and orientation of the writer(s) than about the subject under review (Joyce *et al.*, 1998).

In psychiatry in particular, many individual trials are not large enough to answer the questions we want to answer as reliably as we would want to answer them. Often trials are too small for adequate conclusions to be drawn about potentially small advantages of particular therapies. Advocacy of large trials is a natural response to this situation, but it is not always possible to launch very large trials before therapies become widely accepted or rejected prematurely. In the past the problem has been addressed by the classical narrative review of a set of clinical trials with an accompanying informal synthesis of evidence from the different studies. However, such review articles can, unfortunately, be very misleading as a result of both the possible biased selection of evidence and the emphasis placed upon it by the reviewer to support his or her personal opinion.

An alternative approach that has become increasingly popular in the last decade or so is the *systematic review* which has, essentially, two components:

- *Qualitative*: the description of the available trials, in terms of their relevance and methodological strengths and weaknesses,

- *Quantitative*: a means of mathematically combining results from different studies, even (possibly) when these studies have used different measures to assess the dependent variable.

The quantitative component of a systematic review is usually known as a *meta-analysis*, defined in the *Cambridge Dictionary of Statistics* (Evertt, 2002*b*) as follows:

> A collection of techniques whereby the results of two or more independent studies are statistically combined to yield an overall answer to a question of interest. The rationale behind this approach is to provide a test with more power than is provided by the separate studies themselves.

It is now generally accepted that meta-analysis gives the systematic review an objectivity that is inevitably lacking in literature reviews and can also help the process achieve greater precision and generalizability of findings than any single study. Chalmers and Lau (1993) make the point that both the classical review article and a meta-analysis can be biased, but that at least the writer of a meta-analytic paper is required by the rudimentary standards of the discipline to give the data on which any conclusions are based, and to defend the development of these conclusions by giving evidence that all available data are included, or to give the reasons for not including the data. Chalmers and Lau conclude:

> It seems obvious that a discipline that requires all available data be revealed and included in an analysis has an advantage over one that has traditionally not presented analyses of all the data on which conclusions are based.

The meta-analysis approach, first used as far as we are aware by a psychologist (Glass, 1976), has become increasingly popular in the last decade or so and it is probably fair to say that the majority of statisticians and clinicians are largely enthusiastic about the advantages of meta-analysis over the classical review. But the technique is not without its critics, particularly because of the difficulties of knowing which studies should be included and to which population final results actually apply. Those who remain sceptical do so because they feel that the conclusions from meta-analyses often go beyond what the technique and the data justify, a view nicely summarized in the following quotation from Oakes (1993):

The term meta-analysis refers to the quantitative combination of data from independent trials. Where the results of such combination is a descriptive summary of the weight of the available evidence, the exercise is of undoubted value. Attempts to apply inferential methods, however, are subject to considerable methodological and logical difficulties. The selection and quality of trials included, population bias and the specification of the population to which inference may properly be made are problems to which no satisfactory solutions have been proposed.

Hans Eysenck, one of the earliest critiques of meta-analysis which he believed to be inappropriately combining 'apples' and 'oranges', was, as ever, more pungently critically, using the phrase 'mega silliness' to describe the procedure (Eysenck, 1978).

Despite the concerns expressed by a small number of critics, the demand for systematic reviews of health care interventions has developed rapidly during the last decade, initiated by the widespread adoption of the principles of evidence-based medicine both amongst health care practitioners and policy makers. Such reviews are now increasingly used as a basis for both individual treatment decisions and the funding of health care and health care research worldwide. This growth in systematic reviews is reflected in the current state of the Cochrane Collaboration database containing as it does more than 1200 complete systematic reviews, with a further 1000 due to be added soon.

Systematic reviews have a number of aims:

- to review systematically the available evidence from a particular research area,
- to provide quantitative summaries of the results from each study,
- to combine the results across studies if appropriate; such combination of results leads to greater statistical power in estimating treatment effects,
- to assess the amount of variability between studies,
- to estimate the degree of benefit associated with a particular study treatment,
- to identify study characteristics associated with particularly effective treatments.

Ideally, the trials selected by a systematic review and then subjected to a meta-analysis should be clinically homogeneous. For example, they might all study a similar type of patient for a similar duration with the same treatment in the two arms of each trial. In practice, of course, the trials included are far more likely to differ in some aspects, such as eligibility criterion, duration of treatment, length of follow-up, and how ancillary care is used. On occasions, even treatment itself may not be identical in all the trials. According to Thompson (1998), this implies that, in most circumstances, the objective of a systematic review *cannot* be equated with that of a single large trial, even if that trial has wide eligibility. While a single trial focuses on the effect of a specific treatment in specific situations, a meta-analysis aims for a more generalizable conclusion about the effect of a generic treatment policy in a wider range of areas.

When the trials included in a systematic review do differ in some of their components, therapeutic effects may very well be different, but these differences are likely to be in the *size* of the effects rather than their *direction*. It would, after all, be extraordinary if treatment effects were exactly the same when estimated from trials in different countries, in different populations, in different age groups or under different treatment regimens. If the studies were big enough it would be possible to measure these differences reliably, but in most cases this will *not* be possible. But meta-analysis allows the investigation of sources of possible heterogeneity in the results from different trials as we shall see later, and discourages the common, simplistic, and often misleading interpretation that the results of individual clinical trials are in conflict because some are labelled 'positive' (i.e. statistically significant) and others 'negative' (i.e. statistically non-significant). A systematic approach to synthesizing information can often both estimate the degree of benefit from a particular therapy and whether the benefit depends upon specific characteristics of the studies.

7.2   Study selection

The selection of the studies to be integrated in a systematic review will clearly have a considerable bearing on the conclusions reached. Indeed, according to Pocock (1996), selection of studies is the *greatest* single concern in applying meta-analysis and he identifies three important components of the selection process, *breadth*, *quality* and *representativeness*. Breadth relates to the decision as to whether to study a very specific narrow question (e.g. the same drug, disease and setting for studies following a common protocol) or a more generic problem (e.g. a broad class of treatments for a range of conditions in a variety of settings). Pocock suggests that the broader the meta-analysis, the more difficulty there is in interpreting the combined evidence as regards future policy. Consequently, the broader the meta-analysis the more it needs to be interpreted qualitatively rather than quantitatively.

The representativeness of the studies in a systematic review depends largely on having an acceptable s*earch strategy*. Once the researcher has established the goals of the systematic review, an ambitious literature search needs to be undertaken, the literature obtained, and then summarized. Possible sources of material include the published literature, unpublished literature, uncompleted research reports, work in progress, conference/symposia proceedings, dissertations, expert informants, granting agencies, trial registries, industry and journal hand searching. The search will probably begin by using computerized bibliographic databases of published and unpublished research review articles, for example, MEDLINE. This is clearly a sensible strategy, although there are a number of papers illustrating the deficiencies of MEDLINE searches for randomized controlled trials, see, for example, Bernstein (1988), Gotzsche and Lange (1991), DeNeef (1988) and, more recently, Hopewell *et al.* (2002). The latter reports a comparison of handsearching versus MEDLINE searching to identify reports of randomized controlled trials. A total of 714 reports of randomized trials (as defined by the Cochrane Collaboration) were found by using a combination of handsearching and MEDLINE searching. Of these, 369 (52%) were identified only by handsearching and 32 (4%) were identified only by MEDLINE searching. Of the reports identified only by handsearching, 252 had no MEDLINE record, with 232 of these being meeting abstracts or published in supplements. The remaining 117 papers found only by handsearching were included in the MEDLINE database, but were missed in the electronic search because they did not have either of the publication type terms, 'randomized controlled trial' or 'controlled clinical trial'. Not unreasonably the authors conclude that 'a combination of MEDLINE and handsearching is required to identify adequately reports of randomized trials'. Fortunately help is at hand, since the databases of the two Cochrane Groups that specialize in mental health contain the results of extensive handsearching of a large range of journals, together with regularly updated 'state of the art' electronic searches of numerous databases, and can be readily searched. All trials identified are also located on the Cochrane Database of Clinical Trials.

Finally the quality and reliability of a systematic review is dependent on the quality of the data in the included studies, although criticisms of meta-analyses for including original studies of questionable quality are typical examples of shooting the messenger who bears bad news. Aspects of quality of the original articles that are pertinent to the reliability of the meta-analysis include valid randomization process (we are assuming that in meta-analysis of clinical trials, *only* randomized trials will be selected), minimization of potential biases introduced by dropouts, acceptable methods of analysis particularly in regard to dropouts, level of blinding and recording of adequate clinical details. Several attempts have been made to make this aspect of meta-analysis more rigorous by using the results given by applying specially constructed *quality assessments scales* to assess the candidate trials for inclusion in the analysis. Moher *et al.* (1995), for example, present an annotated bibliography of 25 scales developed to assess quality, all of which the authors consider to have major weaknesses. Consequently it is perhaps not too surprising that the use of such scales in meta-analysis has not been completely successful. Juni *et al.* (1999), for example, used 25 different scales in a meta-analysis of 17 trials comparing low molecular weight heparin with standard heparin for prevention of postoperative thrombosis. They found that for six scales the trials rated as high quality corresponded to those showing no treatment effect, whereas those rated as low quality indicated a significant treatment difference. For another seven scales the reverse was the case. For the remaining 12 scales, effect estimates were similar for those trials rated as high or low quality. In a regression analysis, summary quality scores were not significantly associated with treatment effects. The authors finally concluded that the use of the scales to identify trials of high quality was problematic; instead they recommended that relevant methodological aspects of the trials should be assessed individually and their influence on effect size explored. (Determining quality would be helped if the results from so many trials were not so poorly reported. In the future, this may be improved by the *Consolidation of Standards for Reporting Trials* (CONSORT) statement, Altman *et al.*, 2001, also available at http://consort-statement.org. The core contribution of the CONSORT statement consists of a flow diagram and a checklist both of which are described in Appendix B.)

As an example of how the selection process in a meta-analysis operates in practice we shall use the description provided by Kirsch and Saparstein (1998) in their study of antidepressant medication. Studies assessing the efficacy of antidepressant medication were obtained through a number of previous reviews, supplemented by a computer search of PsycLit and MEDLINE databases from 1974 to 1995 using the search terms, drug therapy or pharmacotherapy or psychotherapy or placebo and depression or affective disorders. Approximately 1500 publications were identified by the literature search. Each of these was examined by one of the authors and those meeting the following criteria were included in the meta-analysis:

- Sample was restricted to patients with a primary diagnosis of depression. Studies were excluded if participants were selected because of other criteria (eating disorders, substance abuse, physical disabilities or chronic medical conditions) as were studies in which the description of the patient population was vague (e.g. 'neurotic').
- Sufficient data were reported or obtainable to calculate within-condition effect sizes. This resulted in the exclusion of studies for which neither pre-post statistical tests nor pre-treatment means were available.
- Data were reported from a placebo control group.
- Participants were between the ages of 18 and 75.

Of the original 1500 studies only 20 met these criteria. Despite the apparent thoroughness of Kirsch and Saparstein's selection procedure, critics of the paper suggested there were flaws and managed to uncover other relevant studies.

7.3 Publication bias

Ensuring that a meta-analysis is truly representative can be problematic. It has long been known that journal articles are not a representative sample of work addressed to any particular area of research (see, for example, Sterlin, 1959; Greenwald, 1975; Smith, 1980). Research with statistically significant results is potentially more likely to be submitted and published than work with null, or non-significant results, particularly if the studies are small (Easterbrook *et al.*, 1991). The problem is made worse by the fact that many medical studies (and this is particular so in psychiatry), look at multiple outcomes, and there is a tendency for only those outcomes suggesting a significant effect to be mentioned when the study is written up. Outcomes that show no clear treatment effect are often ignored, and so will not be included in any later review of studies looking at those particular outcomes. Publication bias is likely to lead to an over representation of positive results.

Clearly it becomes of some importance to assess the likelihood of publication bias in any meta-analysis reported in the literature. A well-known informal method of examining the possibility of publication bias is the so-called *funnel plot*, usually a plot of a measure of a study's precision (for example, one over the standard error), against effect size. The most precise estimates (e.g. those from the largest studies) will be at the top of the plot, and those from less precise or smaller studies at the bottom. The expectation of a 'funnel' shape in the plot relies on two empirical observations:

• The variances of studies in a meta-analysis are not identical, but are distributed in such a way that there are fewer precise studies and rather more imprecise ones.

• At any fixed level of variances, studies are symmetrically distributed about the mean.

Evidence of publication bias is provided by an absence of studies on the left hand side of the base of the funnel. The assumption is that, whether because of editorial policy or author inaction or other reason, these studies (which are not statistically significant) are the ones that might not be published.

To demonstrate how the funnel plot works, Duval and Tweedie (2000) simulated data with zero effect size from 35 hypothetical studies. Figure 7.1 (a) shows the resulting funnel plot; the 95% confidence interval for all 35 studies using the random effects model (see next section) was (−0.18, 0.178), reflecting the true effect size of zero. Next Duval and Tweedie removed the results for the 'left-most' five studies in Fig. 7.1 (a), giving a new funnel plot shown in Fig. 7.1 (b). Again using the

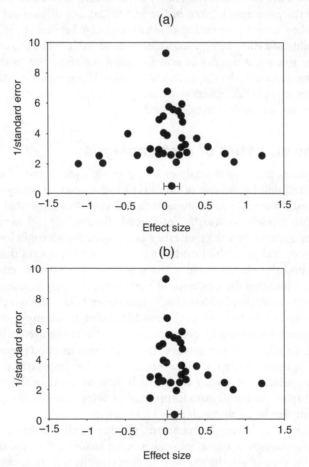

Fig. 7.1 Funnel plots for simulated data (taken with permission from Duval and Tweedie, 2000).

random effect model the 95% confidence interval for those 30 studies was (0.037, 0.210), indicating, incorrectly, a non-zero effect size.

Various suggestions have been made as to how to test for publication bias in a meta-analysis. But the danger of the testing approach is the temptation to assume that, if the test is not significant, there is no problem and the possibility of publication bias can be conveniently ignored. In practice, however, publication bias is very likely endemic to all empirical research and so should be assumed present, whatever the result of some testing procedures with possibly low power.

So rather than simply testing for publication bias, several methods have been proposed for making a suitable 'correction', see, for example, Iyenger and Greenhouse (1988), Silliman (1997a), Givens *et al.* (1997), Taylor and Tweedie (1998), and Copas and Shi (2001). The problem with all of the proposed methods is they make largely unverifiable assumptions, although that by Copas and Shi does appear to be more reasonable than many of the others. A relatively non-technical account of the procedure is given in Everitt (2002a), but its essential feature is a model for the selection process that allows a correlation between the effect size and the probability of a study being selected for meta-analysis. When this correlation is positive the result is a positive bias in the estimated effect size from the meta-analysis. One feature of the Copas and Shi approach that is particularly attractive is the ability to undertake a sensitivity analysis that allows the effect of different amounts of publication bias to be assessed.

7.4 The statistics of meta-analysis

The first aim of many meta-analyses is to provide a global test of significance for the overall null hypothesis of no effect in all studies, or, more commonly, an overall estimate of the magnitude of the effect and an associated confidence interval. Two models are usually considered, *fixed effects* and *random effects*. The former assumes that the true effect is the same for all studies whereas the latter assumes that individual studies have different effect sizes that vary randomly around the overall mean effect size. Thus the random effects model specifically allows for the existence of both between-study heterogeneity and within-study variability. DeMets (1987) and Bailey (1987) discuss the strength and weaknesses of the two competing models. Bailey, for example, suggests that when the research question involves extrapolation to the future—will the treatment have an effect, on the average, then the random effects model for the studies is the appropriate one. The research question implicitly assumes that there is a population of studies from which those analysed in the meta-analysis were sampled, and anticipate future studies being considered or previously unknown studies being uncovered.

When the research question concerns whether treatment has produced an effect, on the average, in the set of studies being analysed, then the fixed effects model for the studies may be the more appropriate; here there is not interest in generalizing the results to other studies.

Many statisticians believe, however, that the random effects model is more appropriate than a fixed effects model for meta-analysis, because between-study variation is an important source of uncertainty that should not be ignored, in assigning uncertainty into pooled results (see, for example, Meier, 1987). A number of authors, for example, Der Simonian and Laird (1986), have suggested conducting a test of homogeneity, i.e. a test that the between-study variance component is zero, and using a fixed effects model if a non-significant result is obtained. Such a test is, however, likely to be of low power for detecting departures from homogeneity and so its practical consequences are probably quite limited.

The technical details of both the fixed and random effects models for meta-analysis are given in Fleiss (1993) and Everitt (2002a) and so are not reported here. The essential feature of both approaches is the use of a weighted mean of treatment effect sizes from the individual studies, with the weights usually being the reciprocals of the associated variances. Effect sizes might be standardized mean differences for continuous response variables, or relative risks or odds ratios for binary outcomes. Both fixed effects and random effects models result in a test of zero effect size and a confidence interval for effect size. But it should be remembered that, in general, a more important aspect of meta-analysis is often the exploration of the likely heterogeneity of effect sizes from the different studies. Random effect models, for example, allow for such heterogeneity but they do not offer any way of exploring and potentially explaining the reasons study results vary. In other words, random effects models do not 'control for', 'adjust for' or 'explain away' heterogeneity.

Understanding heterogeneity should perhaps be the primary focus of the majority of meta-analysis carried out in medicine in general and psychiatry in particular. The examination of heterogeneity may begin with formal statistical tests for its presence, but even in the absence of statistical evidence of heterogeneity, exploration of the relationship of effect size to study characteristics may still be valuable. The question of importance is, what causes heterogeneity in systematic reviews of clinical trials? There are many possible sources of heterogeneity, some of which are essentially *artefactual*, and some of which represent *true* effect modification. Glasziou and Sanders (2002) categorize both potential artefactual and true sources by four factors namely,

- the *patient* or the disease group,
- the *intervention* timing or intensity,
- the *co-intervention*, that is, what other treatments the patient is receiving,
- the *outcome* measurement and timing.

Their conclusions are shown in Table 7.1. Of course, whether heterogeneity is considered artefactual or not is largely a matter of perspective; for example, differences in degree of non-compliance might produce variation in effect sizes that may, in some circumstances, be considered artefactual and in others, an effect modification that has serious policy implications.

Table 7.1 Real and artefactual causes of between-study variation in effect.

	Real	Artefactual
Patient	Disease severity Age Co-morbidity	Improper randomization Differential follow-up (non-comparable groups)
Intervention	Time Duration Dose	Non-compliance Cross-over
Co-intervention	Drugs Therapy	Undetected co-interventions
Outcome	Timing of outcome Event type	Differential and non-differential measurement error

Study of the (possibly) true causes of heterogeneity of treatment effects in a meta-analysis often involves the technique known as *meta-regression* (see, for example, Thompson and Higgins, 2002). Essentially this is nothing more than a weighted regression analysis with effect size as the dependent variable, a number of study characteristics as explanatory variables and weights usually being the reciprocal of the sum of the estimated variance of a study and the estimated between study variance, although other more complex approaches have been described (see, Thompson and Sharp, 1999). Thompson and Higgins (2002) point out that it is important to realize that associations derived from meta-regressions are observational, and have a weaker interpretation than the causal relationships usually inferred from randomized comparisons, particularly when, as is generally the case, averages of patient characteristics in each study are used as the covariates in the regression. Meta-regression can, like subgroup analysis with a single trial, quickly become little more than data dredging. This danger can be partially dealt with at least by pre-specification of the covariates that will be investigated as potential sources of heterogeneity.

To conclude, in our opinion the most important question to ask when contemplating performing a meta-analysis, or reading one, is this question of heterogeneity. Is one comparing like with like, or, in the vernacular, are apples being mixed with oranges? If the answer is yes, then the results of the meta-analysis should be treated with great circumspection, least one fall victim to Eysenck's 'mega silliness'.

7.5 Some examples of meta-analysis of psychiatric trials

In this section we will look at two recent systematic reviews that have been reported in the psychiatric literature, beginning with a study of a well-known alternative therapy that is often suggested as an effective treatment for depression.

7.5.1 Alternative medicine, St John's wort and depression

Magic and medicine have always been closely linked. The African witch doctor, the Native American medicine man, and Europe's medieval alchemist—all were a mixture of magician and physician. All relied heavily on letting a disease run its natural course and the placebo effect for their patients' recovery. Much the same can probably be said about the claims often made for wonderful results from today's alternative medicines—from homeopathy and herbalism to acupuncture and reflexology, therapists continue to earn a good living from a gullible public by pre-empting attempts to subject their treatments to proper scientific investigation using clinical trials with objections such as:

◆ Experience has shown that should there be scepticism and doubt in the mind of a third party close to the patient . . . failure is usually inevitable.

◆ Due to different belief systems and divergent theories about the nature of health and illness, complimentary and alternative medicine disciplines have fundamental differences in how they define target conditions, causes of disease, interventions, and outcome measures of effectiveness.

But in a society as open and susceptible to fraud as ours is, the truth needs all the help it can get, and fortunately some clinicians have taken on the task of evaluating scientifically a number of the more promising alternative therapies, including the use of the herb St John's wort (*Hypericum perforatum*) in the treatment of depression.

Extracts of St John's wort have been used in European folk medicine for centuries and in Germany it has become a mainstream medicine with 20 times more prescriptions written than for Prozac. Anecdotal reports of its effectiveness in treating depressed patients have now been supplemented a number of clinical trials and at least two meta-analyses by Linde *et al.* (1996) and Kim *et al.* (1999). The latter authors, for example, were concerned that earlier studies concluding that St John's wort is an effective antidepressant often employed questionable methodology. In an attempt to correct this, Kim *et al.*, undertook a meta-analysis using only controlled, double-blind studies in which depression was strictly defined. Eligible trials were identified by full text searches in Medline Silver Platter CD-ROM 1983-March 1998 using the following terms:

◆ St John's wort

◆ Hyperic

◆ Alternative medicine

◆ Phytotherapy

◆ Herbal medicine

In addition the authors searched the Psychlit and Psych Index 1987-March 1998, the Internet through different servers, checked bibliographies of obtained articles, and lay publications. To be included in the meta-analysis the studies uncovered had to meet the following three criteria:

- *Design*: Blinded controlled studies that compared St John's wort with placebo or standard antidepressant treatments.
- *Types of participants*: Subjects from similar sociodemographic backgrounds that had depressive disorders defined by either ICD 10, DSM-IIIR, or DSM-IV criteria.
- *Outcome measures*: Clinical outcomes were measured with the Hamilton Depression Scale, a scale known to have high validity and inter-rater reliability.

Six randomized double-blind trials were finally accepted into the meta-analysis. These included 651 patients with mainly mild to moderately severe depressive disorders. Two of the studies were placebo-controlled and the other four compared St John's wort with tricyclic anti-depressant treatments, maprotiline, amitriptyline, and imipramine.

The conclusion of Kim *et al.*'s meta-analysis was that *Hypericum perforatum* was more effective than placebo and similar in effectiveness to low-dose tricyclic antidepressants in the short-term treatment of mild to moderately severe depression, although the authors included a caveat that, despite their stringent selection criteria, serious questions remained regarding the studies analysed. In particular five of the six studies reviewed were carried out in Germany where, as pointed out earlier, St. John's wort is already heavily prescribed for depression. A further limitation was the length of the studies—none of the six trials provided data about long-term outcomes of antidepressant response, side effects, dropout rates, or the rates of relapse for patients on St. John's wort. Finally, in the four trials involving tri-cyclics, what would generally be considered sub-therapeutic doses were used. Kim *et al.* summarized their findings thus:

> Given the current penchant for alternative therapies, St. John's wort could provide the bridge to treatment for those patients that decline conventional antidepressant medications. Future studies, however, need to address the design problems of the current studies before we can conclude that St. John's wort is an effective antidepressant.

Kim *et al.*'s less than enthusiastic endorsement of St John's wort for the treatment of depression, appears to be vindicated by the results from a later trial described in Shelton *et al.* (2001). The authors of the latter were also concerned with the methodological flaws of many of the trials attempting to assess the effectiveness of St John's wort, in particular the failure to use standardized diagnostic practices, resulting in the inclusion of diagnostically heterogeneous groups, and the failure to use standardized rating instruments. In addition Shelton and his co-authors expressed concerns about the relatively short duration of most studies and the possible failure of blinding due to the inability to adequately mask the taste of the St John's wort product. The results of their own randomized, double-blind, placebo-controlled trial involving two hundred adult outpatients concluded that St John's wort was *not* effective for treatment of major depression.

This is therefore a salutary lesson of the dangers of meta analysis. It is only as good as its component parts. A large number of poorly performed, small trials do not add up to the same as a small number, even one, large, well-performed trial. When the two conflict, quality trumps quantity. The St John's Wort story echoes concerns expressed beyond psychiatry. For example, an influential meta-analysis of the use of magnesium in the management of myocardial infarction concluded that it was beneficial. However, when the results of the mega trial that included magnesium were published, it could be clearly seen that it was completely without benefit, and that the smaller studies were flawed. Much the same has happened in the debate about the effects of HRT on the risk of myocardial infarction—in that case meta-analysis of a series of observational studies concluded it was protective—yet the definitive trial not only failed to confirm this, it also raised the possibility that HRT actually increased the risk!

7.5.2 Transcranial magnetic stimulation for depression

Transcranial magnetic stimulation (TMS) involves placing a high intensity magnetic field of brief duration at the scalp surface. This induces an electrical field at the cortical surface that can alter neuronal function. Repetitive TMS (rTMS) involves applying trains of these magnetic pulses. In humans rTMS has been shown to produce changes in frontal lobe blood flow (Teneback et al., 1999) and to normalize the response to dexmethasone in depression (Pridmore, 1999; Ried and Pridmore, 1999). Since trials in the late 1990s, rTMS has been proposed as a treatment for drug resistant depression, schizophrenia and mania (Reid et al., 1998; Pridmore and Belmaker, 1999). McNamara et al. (2001) report a systematic review of the published data, in which randomized controlled trials were searched for using a variety of databases, including MEDLINE and EMBASE. Sixteen published clinical trials of rTMS for depression were identified, but eight were excluded because there was no randomized control group and a further three excluded for reasons given in the original paper. The results from the five trials accepted for the meta-analysis are shown in Table 7.2 (these results are slightly amended from those given in McNamara et al. to enable a simpler investigation of possible publication bias—essentially some zero frequencies have been replaced with a count of one).

Table 7.2 Data for five RCTs of rTMS.

		rTMs	**Placebo**
Trial 1	Improved	11	6
	Not Improved	6	11
Trial 2	Improved	7	1
	Not Improved	1	4
Trial 3	Improved	8	2
	Not Improved	4	4
Trial 4	Improved	4	1
	Not Improved	6	10
Trial 5	Improved	17	8
	Not Improved	18	24

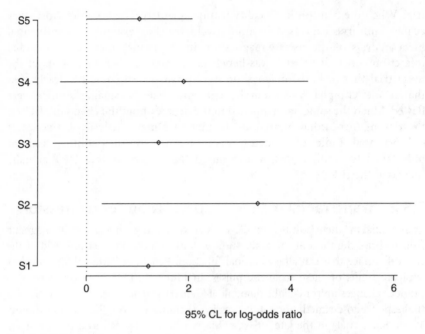

Fig. 7.2 Plot of estimated log-odds ratio and corresponding 95% confidence interval for rTMS trials.

A plot of the estimated log odds ratios from each study and the corresponding 95% confidence intervals is shown in Fig. 7.2. The results appear to be in favour of rTMS. The results from both the fixed effects and random effects model are, for these data, exactly the same. The overall effect size (log odds ratio) is estimated to be 1.33 with a standard error of 0.37, leading to an estimated odds ratio of 3.78 with 95% confidence interval (1.83, 7.81).

For a systematic review that includes so few studies it might be of interest to try to assess the effect of publication bias. Here we apply the procedures proposed by Copas and Shi (2001) and described in less technical terms in Everitt (2002a). Table 7.3 gives the estimated effect size (log odds ratio), associated *P*-value and 95% confidence interval under the possibility of increasing amounts of publication

Table 7.3 Publication bias affect on rTMS meta-analysis.

	Estimated log odds ratio	P-value	95% CI	Number of studies
(Observed data)	1.33	0.003	(0.47,2.19)	5
	1.22	0.017	(0.22, 2.22)	8
	0.73	0.059	(−0.03, 1.48)	12
	0.59	0.332	(−0.60, 1.78)	81

bias. We can see that if the five published studies selected represent only about 50% of the studies carried out, then the effect size becomes non-significant with the confidence interval including the value zero.

7.6 Summary

The systematic review, in particular its quantitative component, meta-analysis, has had a major impact on medical science in the past ten years, and has been largely responsible for the development of evidence-based medical practice. One of the principal reasons that meta-analysis has been so successful is the large number of clinical trials that are now conducted, now of the order of 10 000 per year. Synthesizing results from many studies can be difficult, confusing and ultimately misleading. Meta-analysis has the potential to demonstrate treatment effects with a high degree of precision, possibly revealing small, but clinically important effects. But as with an individual clinical trial, careful planning, comprehensive data collection, and a formal approach to statistical methods is necessary in order to make the results of such an analysis convincing.

Chapter 8

RCTs in psychiatry: Threats, challenges, and the future

8.1 Introduction

In our summary of Chapter 2 of this book, we quoted thus from Palmer (2002):

> Clinical trials are a composite of matters ethical, practical and theoretical. They have had a short but distinguished history, having rapidly become the accepted norm for benchmarking medical progress and yielding the highest quality, single-study evidence for treatment efficacy.

Palmer's glowing commendation of clinical trials is one we heartily endorse, since we are unashamed advocates of the importance of randomized controlled trials for the future of mental health services. We believe they are the best, and often the only, way of deciding what works for whom, and should be the bedrock of any health system serious about improving patient care. But not everybody agrees and our enthusiasm for clinical trials in medicine in general, and psychiatry in particular, is not universally shared. Indeed at the present time, Horton (2001) has declared that 'the accumulated benefits of a half-century of clinical trial research are seriously threatened'. Why?

Possible reasons why clinical trials are currently under threat include:

- Cases both of outright fraud and of trials that have gone wrong have gained wide publicity and produced a public perception that most trials are highly risky and/or ethically dubious.

- Reports of trialists exploiting the vulnerable in poor countries (Rothman and Michels, 2000).

- A minority of clinicians and other experts who continue to question the use of clinical trials in medical research, whose views are widely publicized.

- The increasing suspicion about both the role and the integrity of commercial sponsors of clinical trials, particularly drug trials, funded by pharmaceutical companies.

- The growing demands of twenty-first century patients, who mostly no longer accept the notion of self-sacrifice for the common good, an attitude prevalent at the time of Bradford Hills's early randomized controlled trials (Tudor Hart, 1997). Patients in general do not want to become 'guinea pigs' for the pharmaceutical industry.

◆ The emerging role of patient support groups and the increasing problems of litigation over, for example, informed consent.

Sadly, the vast positive contribution of clinical trials to medicine is mostly hidden from the public eye, and the often lurid journalistic accounts of the few trials that go wrong means that the problems of trials are made all too visible. Horton (2001) suggests that the clinical trial process is approaching a critical moment, with growing public scepticism already producing problems in patient recruitment for some trial organizers. Failure to recruit adequate patient numbers is a real threat to many trials, and often the reason that an unknown number of trials get abandoned and are left unreported.

In this final chapter, we review the objections that have been raised to psychiatric trials in particular. Whilst the reader will not be astonished to learn that we find none of the criticisms to offer fundamental challenges to the use of RCTs in psychiatry, several have some substance, and clearly highlight the inescapable fact that the current practice of clinical trials in psychiatry is far from ideal. Later in the chapter, we will look to the future and consider how the situation can be improved.

8.2 Can randomized clinical trials in psychiatry be justified?

There have been a number of trenchant criticisms of the use of randomized controlled trials to evaluate mental health treatments. It has, for example, been argued that psychiatric treatments are simply too variable and/or too complex to permit generalizations from the particular. An alternative case that has been made is that psychiatric patients are too complex themselves to permit extrapolation from one patient to the wider community. And, of course, there is the continuing claim that the results from most psychiatric trials have little relevance for the day-to-day treatment of the mentally ill, that is the results are not generalizable. Let's consider each of these assertions in turn.

8.2.1 Our interventions are too individual

Psychiatry is not 'cook book' medicine. One of the things that most appealed to one of us when contemplating clinical training in psychiatry was the importance given to the detailed assessment of virtually every aspect of a patient's life and background when assessing the patient's condition. Even diagnosis was not the 'open and shut' case that it had been in clinical medicine, with often complex formulations being preferred to stark statements such as 'this patient has cancer of the lung'. Likewise, treatments, or more particularly, the 'talking treatments', were more subtle, more considered and, even sometimes more complicated, than the pharmaceutical circus of modern cardiology.

We must therefore consider seriously the charge that the same diversity that makes psychiatry or psychology both fascinating and challenging, means that the RCT is both inappropriate and inadequate for assessing our success or failure in treatment. For example, taking one voice from many, Silberschatz articulates the principal arguments against RCTs in psychiatry from the perspective of a psychotherapist (Persons and Silberschatz, 1998). For him, the important questions are: what is bothering the patient? What do they hope to achieve? Why have they not achieved that? And so on and so forth. The argument continues that manualization, deemed essential in psychological treatment trials to enable another clinician to be able to repeat the intervention later, and to ensure that the therapy is replicable, removes the heart of psychological treatment—empathy, therapeutic alliance, and so on. For critics of the RCT like Silberschatz (and he is certainly not a lone voice), what is lost is the essential individual nature of psychological treatments. People are different, problems are different, and therefore, the argument goes, so should the treatments be different.

But this debate is not unique to psychiatry; very similar questions are raised by those sceptical of the place of clinical trials in the assessment of alternative or complementary medicine (see Mason *et al.*, 2002). Once again, it is claimed that the 'human experience' is central to the treatment process, and that the treatment is really part of a complex patient–practitioner interaction; outcomes, such as personal growth or spiritual gain, are not easily measured. More problematic is the thorny question of expectation, namely, that someone who attends a particular complementary practitioner's has a strong belief in the treatment under offer, and that such credibility and expectation of therapeutic gain will bias the results of any trials, particularly if, as in psychotherapy trials, the treatment cannot be blinded.

How can we counter such arguments against trying to evaluate psychiatric treatments scientifically via RCTs? It is, of course, true that people are different, but this applies across medicine. Our caricature of medicine given above is exactly that, a caricature. A cardiologist who fails to notice that people differ even if ventricles do not (and we are prepared to accept that even ventricles differ!) would be a poor cardiologist indeed. A hundred or so years of writing on the 'art of medicine', the recent growth of 'narrative based medicine', and the seemingly endless critiques of the limitations, or at least the perceived limited scope, and indeed limited success of narrowly orientated biomedicine, show that across the entire medical profession, no one should seriously dispute the importance of understanding the individual.

But if that was all there was, if every patient was indeed unique and every problem without precedent, then medicine in general and psychiatry in particular would come to a full stop. If there were no commonalities between our patients, and no identifiable general patterns in particular groups of patients, then there would be no purpose in medical education, or any purpose in clinical experience and training. It is these shared factors that permit clinicians to draw on what they have learnt both from their training and their experience, and then use this acquired knowledge to assess and understand the specific patient now requiring their attention. After all, an intelligent being cannot treat every person (or every object) it sees as a unique entity;

rather it has to classify patterns and information so that it may apply its hard-won knowledge about similar people encountered in the past, to the person at hand.

And it is the existence of patterns of disease that make clinical trials viable. Having observed some phenomenon previously in a patient population of interest, be it a certain cancer, a particularly behaviour, a biochemical abnormality, or an emotional reaction, means that there is something that might form the basis for a clinical trial. The systematically acquired information that results can be used to help future patients, without forgetting that what is truly unique about a patient (and so cannot be studied in a clinical trial), still has to be taken into account in caring for the patient, and for this, the treating clinician will often need large amounts of intuition, experience, and empathy.

8.2.2 Our patients are too complex

Psychiatric disorders are frequently not straightforward, and psychiatric patients often display challenging and complex behaviours that might, at first sight, appear incompatible with the tightly controlled demands of most clinical trials. Broad categories such as depression or schizophrenia hide several sub groups, whose boundaries are imperfectly delineated. Many (perhaps most) psychiatric patients have more than one diagnosis, something that has come to be labelled as *comorbidity*. What use is it studying those rare patients in whom depression does not co-exist with other disorders, such as anxiety or substance abuse, when in 'real life' these so often go together? And is it really possible to recruit members of 'difficult' patient populations and to maintain them in a trial according to the often, stringent requirements of the trial protocol?

Complications of diagnosis and patient complexity can both be difficult challenges to be faced by psychiatric trialists, but neither provides *fundamental* objections to the use of RCTs in psychiatry. Comorbidity may, for example, affect generalization, if the index trial was performed on an unusually 'pure' subgroup of patients, but the validity of the data is unaffected. And trials can be (and have been) conducted, and conducted to a high standard, in populations and situations that might seem insuperable to the faint hearted. Schizophrenia and substance abuse, for example, does not seem an auspicious subject for an RCT, since patients with both problems ('dual diagnosis' in the jargon), are sometime seen as 'unascertainable, unconsentable, untreatable and untrackable'. But a research group in Manchester in the UK performed just such a trial to good effect (Barrowclough *et al.*, 2001). Again it might be predicted that it would be impossible to carry out randomized trials in violent forensic patients, yet there is a seminal trial in which 321 mentally disordered offenders were randomly assigned to either release or outpatient compulsory treatment (Swartz *et al.*, 2001).

8.2.3 Our interventions are too complex

In effect, this is much the same argument as in the previous sections, namely, that psychiatry is too individual a subject, and that far too many things happen during even a single consultation, to permit evaluation by the technology of the RCT.

Certainly, many of the interventions that have been developed for the treatment of mental health problems are more complex than drug treatments. Some characteristics of such complex interventions that are thought by some to raise doubts about the suitability of clinical trials for their evaluation, are identified by Crawford *et al.* (2002):

• Complex interventions comprise multiple inter-connecting elements.

• Complex interventions have mechanisms of action that are difficult to identify.

• Complex interventions have effects that depend on a range of factors, including the actions of the practitioners who deliver them.

But no one has ever claimed that the RCT can tell you everything about psychiatry and the complexities of treatment. And so long as any intervention can be adequately described and reproduced, easy for a single drug, more difficult but certainly achievable for a psychological treatment, then that intervention can be scrutinized by a clinical trial.

Although we do not accept that our interventions are inherently too complex to be assessed by randomized clinical trials, we readily concede that in mental health we seem to have a vested interest in making things more complex than necessary. Diagnostic issues in psychiatry, for example, can become something of a fetish, and taken to extremes can undermine the inherent simplicity of the clinical trial; few clinicians really care, for example, about the sub divisions of somatoform disorders or whether someone has dysthymia or double depression. And psychiatrists use far too many rating scales to measure far too many things in their trials, increasing the chances of false positive findings (as the Oxford, UK, group of trialists note, 'many trials would be of much greater scientific value if they collected 10 times less data on 10 times more patients'). An analysis of trials on the Cochrane Schizophrenia Data base found that over 640 different rating scales had been employed (Thornley *et al.*, 1998; Gilbody *et al.*, 2002). The use of a large number of outcome measures is driven by the fear of missing something that might be 'clinically significant', even if that 'something' was not the primary reason for carrying out the study. But any advantages of such an approach are massively outweighed by the disadvantages, in particular those of multiple testing, and the loss of simplicity, both in analysis and in understanding of results.

8.2.4 The results are not generalizable

In Chapter 4, we discussed the question of explanatory versus pragmatic trials. We suggested there that the current vogue for pragmatic trials arises from the perception that many explanatory clinical trials take place in 'pure' populations, for example, those free from all forms of comorbidity, with participants keen to attend follow-ups, happy to take medication, and so on and so forth, with the consequence that the results were not considered relevant to the vast majority of the population who *do* suffer from comorbidity, and who are, in general, reluctant to do any of the things mentioned. Likewise, prognostic features of patients in clinical trials may vary, even within trials, and it is certainly true that one cannot assume that because a treatment has been successful in a well-conducted clinical trial, the results will apply to all patients with the same diagnosis (Rothwell, 1995).

Our conclusion in Chapter 4 was that there is much merit in the arguments for more pragmatic trials in psychiatry. Indeed, we would agree with other commentators that the main criticism that can be sustained against the RCT in psychiatry, as currently undertaken, is the issue of generalizability (McKee *et al.*, 1999). But note the rider, 'as currently undertaken'. The fault lies not with the principles of the randomized clinical trial, but simply the way such trials are often conducted at present. The answer, as we will discuss later, is not for psychiatry to turn its back on the RCT, but for trialists to push for larger, simpler trials, and to lobby against the increasing bureaucratization of the clinical trial that stands in the way of achieving these objectives.

8.3 Are randomized clinical trials really necessary?

One further objection still occasionally raised about clinical trials is randomization, a debate considered in detail in Chapter 2. Readers will recall that there are some common sense situations when it is clearly unethical to randomize, namely when that would deprive a trial participant of a treatment that is *known* to be effective. The reader will also recall our strong conviction that there are more situations in clinical practice when it is unethical *not* to randomize rather than the converse. Nevertheless, attempts have been made to lessen the random allocation component of clinical trials, and a number of these, for example, patient preference trials, were discussed in Chapter 3.

But there remain some voices opposed to *all* forms of randomized clinical trials, on the essentially pragmatic grounds, that they consider non-randomized studies perfectly adequate to answer the questions generally posed about the effectiveness of treatments, within perhaps a less artificial framework than the clinical trial, and certainly with less cost and effort. Recent support for such a point-of-view comes from two papers in the prestigious *New England Journal of Medicine*, both claiming to show that the results of observational trials matched those of RCTs of the same intervention for the same conditions (Concato *et al.*, 2000; Benson *et al.*, 2000). The implication of the findings (if true) from these two papers is why should anybody bother undertaking a randomized clinical trial if the indisputably easier and cheaper to perform observational study gives the same answer anyway?

The problem is, of course, that the results given in Concato (2000) and Benson (2000), contradict many other reports in the literature that have found that non-randomized studies yield larger estimates of treatment effects than studies that use random allocation, estimates that are very likely biased. Examples are the investigations reported in Chalmers *et al.* (1977), Sacks *et al.* (1983), Spilker (1991) and Kunz & Oxman (1998). In Spilker's book, for example, there is a review of the results from non-randomized trials and randomized trials in four major clinical areas; one of these is psychiatry and Spilker finds that 83% of non-randomized studies reported positive findings, as compared to only 25% of RCTs. Certainly, the majority of the research community, which greeted the papers by Concato *et al.* (2002) and Benson (2002) with 'uproar' (Barton, 2000), like the authors of this book remain totally unconvinced of the equivalence of randomized and non-randomized trials. The evidence that non-randomized trials (and randomized trials with inadequately concealed allocation—see Schultz *et al.*, 1995) result, on average, in overestimates of effect size seems overwhelming (a further recent confirmation that this is the case is provided by Kunz *et al.*, 2002).

It is of course possible that, as Cancato and Benson suggest, observational studies have improved over the years, but we are sceptical that this has happened to any meaningful extent, sufficient to remove the inherent biases in such studies. It is more likely, as the critics of the two papers have suggested, that the trials selected by the authors for the comparison were from an atypical, selected group (Barton, 2000; Pocock and Elbourne, 2000). Since then, the vehement debates on the effectiveness of screening to reduce mortality from breast cancer, and of HRT to prevent heart attacks, both supported by observational data but not RCTs, remind us that the position of the randomized controlled clinical trial at the head of the 'evidence hierarchy' remains fully justified.

Of course, observational studies can be important in many circumstances, and provide much useful information. For example, a study of the effect of training of the ability of Dutch general practitioners to recognize and treat depression used a before and after design—the intervention was associated with an improvement in the management of depression in the short term, but by the end of the study no effects were detected, Tiemens *et al.* (1999). Because the overall results were negative, the study did generate useful information. We cannot be sure that the intervention produced even the short-term benefits, since there is no way one can adjust for other factors, such as changes in the health care system, or the appearance of new treatments, but if the intervention was successful, we can infer that its effect was anyway not long lasting.

8.4 The future of psychiatric trials

An optimist is someone who thinks the future is uncertain. Anon.

What does the future hold for clinical trials in psychiatry? Should we be optimistic or pessimistic? Psychiatrists have the reputation in medical circles of never answering a straight question, and eternally fence sitting (in this respect at least, psychiatrists and statisticians seem to suffer from the same malaise). We regret that we are going to conform to this stereotype, since we are simultaneously both optimistic and pessimistic about the future. But before coming to the reasons for this uncertainty, let's examine what we anticipate for psychiatric trials in the coming years:

◆ The current move towards larger, simpler trials will accelerate and would be welcome. However, it is likely that the increasing bureaucratization of trials, with directive piling on directive, will mitigate against this.

- There will be greater 'consumer' (a word we dislike) involvement in setting priorities. This is to be welcomed, not least if it leads to a demystification of clinical trials, and a shared understanding of their role in protecting patients from untried and untested therapies. It will also mean a greater willingness to mix assessments methods—for example, incorporating a greater use of *qualitative methods* (Crawford *et al.*, 2002). Such methods may help to identify the cultural context, values, beliefs, and community norms of target groups, and thus provide the key to the designing and the implementation of promising interventions (see Stephenson & Imrie, 1998).

- The assessment of complex interventions, such as new services, or combinations of drugs, psychotherapy, and social interventions, will become more prominent. More sophisticated methodologies will need to be developed to assess these, albeit not departing from the fundamental principle of the RCT, which, as we never tire of repeating, is to abolish selection bias from unmeasured factors of possible or probable prognostic importance. However, there is a clear role for incorporating qualitative research methods into the experimental evaluation. For example, we agree with the recommendations of a recent National Institutes of Health committee, that more attention should be paid to issues such as the representativeness of recruitment, values, and preferences of trial participants, and broader outcome measures (functioning, work and so on, rather than symptoms alone).

- Promising new interventions are likely to appear from unexpected quarters. Although we do not see this as posing any unique challenges, just continued investment in the infrastructure and training is needed to assess them.

At the top of our own particular 'wish list' for the future of psychiatric trials, we place size, simplicity, and realism. Make psychiatric trials 'bigger' (larger numbers of patients), 'simpler' (less outcome measures, for example), and more 'life like' (in psychiatry, perhaps more so than any other discipline, the case for more pragmatic trials of what we actually do is compelling). Since we have largely dealt with the 'simpler' and the 'life-like' in other chapters, let's concentrate here on the 'bigger'.

As we have constantly made clear throughout this book, we are unashamed advocates of the clinical trial. We have heard no compelling arguments as to why randomized clinical trials should yet be replaced at the top of the hierarchy of medical evidence when evaluating the effectiveness of treatment, a position given to them nearly 30 years ago by Byar (1978)—see Table 8.1. But clinical trials can, of course, give results that are shown eventually as very likely to have been wrong. Clinical trials can and do give answers, that in retrospective are seen to have been in error. It is easy to see this when trials report positive results of treatments, only to be followed by later RCTs that find them ineffective, or which are anyway implausible. One example of this happening was provided in Chapter 7, in our discussion of trials investigating the effectiveness of St John's Wort. A further example (one that may possibly offend a small number of readers), involves the existence of many positive trials of homeopathy, allied to (at least to our way of thinking) the compelling arguments that homeopathy cannot 'work' in any accepted sense of the word (other than as a placebo).

Table 8.1 Hierarchy of Medical Evidence (from Byar, 1978).

- ◆ Case reports
- ◆ Case series
- ◆ Database studies
- ◆ Observational studies
- ◆ Controlled clinical trials
- ◆ Randomized controlled trial

So, in what circumstances are clinical trials most likely to give 'wrong' answers? There are many reasons, largely methodological, but we choose to focus on the issue we think the most paramount—that of size. Clinical trials may give results that are later seen as flawed, simply because they were too small and small trials can only detect large effects. But large treatment effects, unless one has stumbled on the next penicillin, are usually *a priori* implausible. Instead, most advances in medicine and psychiatry are incremental, involving small but important advances, rather than earth shattering breakthroughs. 'Moderate (but worthwhile) effects on major outcomes are generally more plausible than large effects' (Collins *et al.*, 1996).

The name of the game across medicine is therefore detecting small, but reasonable effects. But what constitutes reasonable? In the United Kingdom, the influential Oxford Group of researchers gives an instructive example. A single treatment might reduce the risk of death after heart attacks from 10 per 100 patients to 8 or 9. This might not seem very much, and would make little difference to the chances of survival of any single patient. But taken world-wide, this would prevent 10 000 to 20 000 premature deaths, a very dramatic decrease, that result because heart attacks are common, so a small reduction in risk has a large effect on the population (Collins *et al.*, 1996).

The problem is that a modest risk is likely to be hidden in most small trials, simply as a result of the vagaries of chance, or modest or even relatively small biases. Clearly making sure a trial is run to high standards, with good allocation concealment, few losses to follow up and an intention to treat analysis will help, but realistically the approach most likely to provide an answer that is a close approximation to the truth is a large trial.

The example we quoted above comes from cardiology, and this is not accidental, since it was in cardiology that the first 'mega trials' were undertaken. One of us (SW) can well remember working on the Coronary Care Unit at Oxford when the first such trial, known as ISIS, was underway, although he was blithely unaware of the significance of what was happening, merely irritated by the constant phone calls coming to the Unit from round the world to receive the randomization codes! That trial was the first in a series of genuinely epoch-making trials that have transformed the treatment of myocardial infarction. The same author's father also took part in the fourth such trial—this time as one of 58 050 patients (Isis-4, 1995)!

Moving on from cardiology to a more pertinent situation (at least for this book) of mental health, let us take the example of antidepressants. The management of depression is a fundamental question for psychiatry. At present, there is no doubt that there are two classes of drugs, the tricyclics and their newer rivals, the selective serotonin reuptake inhibitors (SSRIs) both effective in management. But which is better? And what does 'better' mean?

We might easily agree that should one class of drugs be, say 50%, better (however defined) than the other, then this group would immediately become the treatment of choice and the results would represent a dramatic breakthrough in treatment. Even a 25% improvement in outcome from one class of antidepressants over the other would be of considerable importance, and indeed still be close to being a 'dramatic breakthrough'. But since depression is a very common problem worldwide (the World Bank analysis predicts that it will be the second most common cause of disability across the world by 2020), most psychiatrists would agree that even a 10% improvement produced by one class of drugs over the other would be a very worthwhile benefit.

Sadly, the evidence from the literature of trials comparing tricyclics with SSRIs demonstrates that such trials were incapable of detecting any difference much smaller than the 'dramatic breakthrough'. Hotopf and colleagues (Hotopf *et al.*, 1997), for example, analyzed all the trials that compared tricyclics 'head to head' with SSRIs (there were 121 of them at the time of the study—there are probably more today). Quite a few of the trials were sufficiently large to be able to detect that SSRIs were about 50% better in improving outcome than tricyclics; none of course did, and such a quantum leap in efficacy was always improbable. But we have argued that if the SSRIs were actually 20% better, this would be real progress and worthwhile knowing. Less than a dozen of the trials of those examined by Hotopf *et al.* (1997) could have detected such an effect. And if the differences were 10%—perhaps the most realistic possibility, then not a single trial could have come anywhere near detecting what would still be an important improvement in the management of depressed patients, although, of course, systematic reviews and meta analyses could assist.

(Since the publication of the Hotopf *et al.* paper, the sample size of antidepressant trials has indeed started to increase—for example, Kurt Kroenke and colleagues in the United States carried out a study designed to directly compare three antidepressants, and this time used a sample size of 573 adult depressed patients recruited from primary care, Kroenke *et al.*, 2001. They also failed to find any differences, but for the first time we can be more confident that had important differences existed, this study would have had the power to detect them.)

So that it appears that trials in depression are seriously under-powered for detecting small but important differences between treatments, and the situation is no better in schizophrenia. For example, a study of over 2000 trials in schizophrenia found that the mean sample size was about 60 (Thornley, 1998). And although Johnson (1998) from a search of the four leading psychiatric journals from 1956 to 1996 found that the number of patients per treatment group in psychiatric trials was indeed rising over the four decades, the increase, from 17 to 25 over 40 years, was hardly impressive (Johnson, 1998)!

Fortunately, there are now some encouraging signs of change. As far as we know, the largest trial yet completed in psychiatry is the Lilly sponsored study comparing olanzapine with haloperidol, for the treatment of schizophrenia, which randomized 1996 patients across Europe and North America (Tollefson *et al.*, 1997)—although the amount of information collected means that by no stretch of imagination could it be called a 'simple' trial—it cost $55 million dollars, collected vast quantities of data on each participant, and perhaps as a result had a high attrition rate. At the same time, researchers in the United Kingdom completed what may be the largest trial looking at different models of community care—the so-called 'UK 700' study which actually recruited 708 patients (UK 700 Group: Creed, 1999). And in progress, as we write, is what could have been the largest trial yet seen in psychiatry, since the initial aim was to recruit 3000 patients with a diagnosis of bipolar affective disorder to provide a comparison of lithium, valproate, and a combination of the two (Geddes, 2002). Sadly, problems with funding meant that the sample size had to be reduced to 1068, but the final study will still be a major contribution. We wish them luck.

The case for large-scale trials in psychiatry seems compelling. But sadly (and paradoxically), the current climate is becoming less friendly to such trials. For a large trial to have any chance of success, it needs to have very simple methodology, to involve as little disruption to normal clinical care as possible, to involve collecting the least amount of data that is required, to recruit patients as close to 'real life' as possible, and to have simple, streamlined consent procedures. Unfortunately, the seemingly endless series of directives from Trusts, the Department of Health, regulatory bodies and the European Union, all seem to be moving in the other direction. Geddes and his co-workers, for example, note how the current fashions for restrictive entry criteria, excessive concern with minor diagnostic issues, elaborate consent procedures often having to be repeated 24 hours later, excessive collection of data that may never be used (all those quality of life and economic measures, for example), and excessive auditing of data to detect minor and inconsequential errors, all are inimical to large-scale trials.

Large trials are urgently necessary in psychiatry but are not a panacea for all ills. They are costly in terms of resource and time. They have to be simple, yet as we have heard, psychiatric interventions are not necessarily simple (it is all very well to carry out a mega trial of aspirin, but we doubt there would have been the same enthusiasm for a similarly large trial of, for example, aortic valve surgery). In most large trials the intervention itself is of relatively short duration, sometimes just a single tablet—but this is unlikely to be the case in psychiatry.

So it remains important to strike a balance between the desire for large trials and what is possible, given the probable financial and temporal constraints. Yes, as standard treatments improve, we need to work towards detecting smaller, but still important, treatment effects using a single large trial. But many trials in psychiatry will remain under-powered, and so we will continue to require the systematic and the statistical assessments of several smaller trials to answer particular questions. Quality will, of course, always be demanded, whatever the size of the trial.

8.5   Defending the clinical trial

The editor of the *Lancet*, Richard Horton, a powerful advocate of modern medicine's need for securing high-quality evidence, gave a keynote address at the 2001 *Society for Clinical Trials* annual meeting, provocatively entitled, 'The clinical trial: deceitful, disputable, unbelievable, unhelpful, and shameful-what next?' Each adjective in the title was supported by evidence from examples. Horton's intention was to confront trialists with the likely consequences of clinical trials, if considerable effort is not made soon to improve the public image of such studies and make the public more aware of their importance. In the 'What Next' section of his paper, Horton proposes four possible lines of action:

- Those who take part in clinical trials must become more powerful advocates for those trials. The hidden benefits of clinical trials must be no longer hidden. There needs to be a more concerted effort to help the public understand how biases and the play of chance can lead to dangerously incorrect conclusions about the effects of healthcare interventions.

- Trialists must show greater concern for the threatened integrity of the clinical trial process. Reporting instances of proven misconduct, as soon as they come to light, is part of the scientist's responsibility to patients.

- Researchers need to think more critically about the practical methodology of the studies they undertake. Action is needed to promote awareness of randomized trials underway, to ensure that trials address issues of importance, are acceptable to patients and clinicians, and that practical support is provided for participating centres. An emphasis on the better care a patient receives in a clinical trial would be one way ahead (see Chapter 2).

- More attention needs to be given to the process of informed consent, which is the ethical *sine qua non* of clinical trials. Details of the potential benefits and risks of the study need to be as transparent and honest as possible, particularly with the increasing possibility of medical malpractice lawsuits being filed against trial sponsors if things go wrong.

Horton sums up his recommendations thus:

> All health-care professionals directly or peripherally involved in clinical trials need to recommit themselves to explaining, proselytising, promoting, understanding, encouraging, studying, protecting, strengthening, and reflecting on the clinical trial process.

8.6   Summary

Early in this book, we implied that no satisfactory alternative exists to the randomized controlled trial for evaluating competing therapies. Having now described the alternatives in the intervening chapters, we hope that readers will largely agree with our conclusion that randomization is far and away the most satisfactory way of deciding if one treatment if more effective than another in dealing with a particular condition. 'All things being equal, randomised controlled trials are more able to attribute effects to causes' (Barton, 2000) remains our motto.

But as Archie Cochrane once said, 'The randomised controlled trial is a very beautiful technique of wide applicability, but as with everything else there are snags.' Clinical trials are certainly not perfect but they remain the essential methodology in the evaluation of the effectiveness of treatments. No alternative is available that is more likely to give results that will lead to confident recommendations about treating patients that can be used to improve clinical care. But currently, there is a worrying imbalance in the public perception of clinical trials; clinical trials are associated with perceptions of risk, danger, fraud, misconduct, exploitation, rather than being regarded as a major contributor to improvements in health and well-being. There is a very real danger that a growth in scepticism about trials, allied to the growing network of concerned patient support groups, will eventually prevent adequate patient recruitment in many proposed trials. And today's patients, whether members of support groups or not, have high expectations and are better informed, largely due to the unprecedented amounts of information available via the Internet. They are more likely to question clinicians about procedures such as blinding, placebos, and randomization, and will need convincing answers if they are to agree to participate in any proposed trial.

The challenge for trialists in the future is to convince an increasingly well-informed public that randomized clinical trials are necessary and valuable, and that discarding this methodology will likely lead to confusion regarding the value of treatments, and to worthless and dangerous treatments becoming prevalent. Trialists will need to take the public with them. Trials need to be represented not as experiments to be carried out on patients, but as collaborations between trialists and patients. The clinical trial researcher of the future will have to be not just an expert in methodology, etc. but also an advocate. Those who carry out clinical trials must become better and more passionate activists for trials, prepared to defend their case passionately in order to persuade both the public and the professionals of its strength. If they can, then the clinical trial, whilst it will not be totally unchanged and unchallenged, will likely remain the gold standard for evaluating new treatments for the foreseeable future. If they cannot, then the future for clinical trials is likely to be gloomy. The authors of this book remain very firmly attached to their fence.

Appendix A

Issues in the management of clinical trials—'how to do it'

A1   Introduction

What follows is intended as a practical guide to the day-to-day business of developing, funding and managing a clinical trial. As in so much in life, the devil is in the details, and there will be a considerable amount of work to be done before any trial gets under way, with participants being recruited and data collected. Well before this happens (if it ever does!) the investigators will need to choose the right question and make sure the proposed study is needed. Most grant giving bodies now formally require evidence of a systematic review before funding a new trial. After all, there is no point in attempting to answer a question if it has already been answered. At this stage it is sufficient to consult publically available databases such as the Cochrane Library to assess the current state of knowledge. If there has been a Cochrane Review in the area that it is hoped to investigate, quote it, and also take particular note of the conclusions, including the 'Recommendations for Future Research'. It is also helpful to consult registers of existing clinical trials, such as *www.controlled-trials.com*. Following these initial steps it may be helpful to produce a one- or two-page document describing the essential scientific and clinical features of the proposed study and use this to gather feedback from experts not in the trial team. Any worthwhile ideas and suggestions arising from this process can then be used to amend the original plan before investing the considerable time needed to produce perhaps the most important document in launching a clinical trial, the *trial protocol*.

A2   Clinical trial protocols

All clinical trials begin with a document that specifies the research plan for the trial. This document is known as the trial protocol. The protocol serves as a guide for the conduct of the trial and must describe in a clear and unambiguous manner how the trial is to be performed, so that all the investigators associated with the trial are familiar with the procedures to be used. The trial protocol must summarize published work on the study topic and use the results from such work to justify the need for the trial. If drugs are involved, then pertinent pharmacological and toxicity data should be included. The purpose of the trial and its current importance need to be described in clear and concise terms. Hypotheses that the trial is designed to test need to be clearly specified and the population of patients to be entered into the trial fully described. The protocol must specify the treatments to be used; in particular, for drug studies, the dose to be administered, the dosing regimen, and the duration of dosing all need to be listed. Details of the randomization scheme to be adopted must be made explicit in the protocol along with other aspects of design such as control groups, blinding, sample size determination and the number of interim analyses planned (if any).

According to Piantadosi (1997) the protocol is the single most important control tool for all aspects of a clinical trial, because it contains a complete specification for both the research plan and treatment for the individual patient. The protocol serves several purposes:

♦ It provides an effective method of communicating research ideas and plans in detail to other investigators.

♦ For regulatory bodies the protocol is a legal document in addition to its other functions.

♦ The protocol specifies all aspects of the statistical design of a clinical trial so that the quantitative conclusions of the study are conditional upon it.

♦ The protocol is often the document used in efforts to procure funding for the trial.

♦ The protocol (and associated information and consent forms) provides the material both for peer review of an intended trial and examination of the trial's ethical and legal implications by the appropriate ethical committee(s).

All of these functions need to be kept in mind when preparing the trial protocol, and the document needs to give a clear and pertinent definition of the project particulars when it is used in seeking funds for the trial.

There is no such thing as a master plan for writing a universal trial protocol applicable in all circumstances (some useful references are Spilker, 1984; Collins, 1998). Nevertheless, there is enough common ground to provide some very useful guidelines. The protocol needs to be written in a structured formal style with page numbers and references. The key headings for the majority of protocols will include most of the following:

♦ **Title page**. Title, head investigator, co-investigators, supporting organizations, all relevant addresses and telephone numbers. For some trials it may also be necessary to provide curriculum vitae for the main investigators.

♦ **Synopsis/Abstract**. A short (one page or less) describing the rationale, objectives and significance of the trial, along with a summary of the treatments to be used, the patient population to be studied, the number of patients to be recruited and the primary outcome measures.

◆ **Schema**. A table or graph describing patient recruitment to the trial and flow through the trial; the aim is to allow the basic structure of the trial to be visible relatively simply, without the details of therapy, doses, schedules, etc.

◆ **Background**. This section provides the scientific background for the study and should be such that it can be read and understood by other researchers and reviewers who are not as expert in the particular area of the study as the trial investigators themselves. References should be included and the aim in this section should be a narrative style. Any unpublished work that the investigators have done on the subject of the trial should be described here.

◆ **Details of objectives**. Here both the main and secondary (if any) objectives of the trial need to be stated clearly and concisely, and the hypotheses to be tested by the study spelt out in detail. Reasons for carrying out the trial need to be made clear; for example, to test a new treatment regimen, or to determine the best of a number of current standard treatments.

◆ **Drug information**. For drug trials the compounds to be used need to be specified, along with information about toxicity, stability, supplier, etc.

◆ **Inclusion and exclusion criteria**. A detailed specification of participants who are eligible and those who are considered ineligible for the trial. For example, if the trial is investigating a new treatment for male schizophrenics under the age of 50, the inclusion criteria might specify that patients be (i) male, (ii) <50 years of age with (iii) a diagnosis of schizophrenia. Remember that having a large number of inclusion and exclusion criteria may ensure a more homogeneous trial population, but it may also make the results from the trial less generalizable, as well as making patient recruitment more difficult.

◆ **Subject withdrawal criteria**. When and how to withdraw participants from the trial and the type and timing of the data to be collected for withdrawn subjects.

◆ **Treatment**. Specify the treatment, formulation, dosage, dosing regimen, duration of treatments both active and placebo. Procedures for monitoring the compliance of participants need to be specified. Specific details of complex interventions should usually be described in an appendix or in a separate training manual.

◆ **Randomization scheme**. Details of the type of randomization to be used and the procedures for both maintaining and, when necessary, breaking randomization codes. Any strata identified (see Chapter 3) to ensure that treatment assignments are equally distributed over important prognostic factors need to be detailed.

◆ **Outcome measures**. The details of both the primary and secondary (if any) outcome variables to be used in the study, particularly those designed to assess treatment efficacy, along with the proposed schedule of when the measurements and observations are to be made.

◆ **Power/sample size calculations**. Details of how the number of subjects to be recruited into the sample was determined, including the power to be achieved, the treatment effect size used, and the variance assumed for the primary outcome. And remember no one will believe a protocol that states that a single investigator is going to personally recruit dozens or even hundreds of patients. In such cases you will need collaborators.

◆ **Data recording, management and monitoring**. Details of how data is to be collected and its quality ensured during the trial.

◆ **Statistical analysis**. A description of the statistical methods to be employed, including timing of any planned interim analyses. When the data to be collected is longitudinal, procedures for dealing with dropouts need to be made clear, as does the method of analysis to be used. Mention of the software to be used is often helpful.

◆ **Adverse effects**. Specify how adverse effects are to be detected and recorded, and the names and addresses of persons to be contacted in case of severe adverse effects.

◆ **Publications**. Indicate the form in which the results of the trial will be reported (official report, scientific article, etc.).

◆ **Study budget/insurance/financial sources**. Give details of how the trial is funded and how the money is to be allocated.

(In the United Kingdom the *Medical Research Council* (MRC) which funds many trials in psychiatry have a proforma that mandates certain headings—see *MRC Guidelines for Good Clinical Practice in Clinical Trials*: www.mrc.ac.uk. These can be downloaded in electronic form and provide useful guidelines for writing a protocol even when making an application for funding to some other body.)

Having written the protocol it may be helpful to develop partnerships with user groups, invite their comments on the protocol and budget for their ongoing input. Indeed, in the future this seems likely to be mandatory—the current Research Governance Framework for NHS Research states that 'Users are to be involved, as appropriate, in the development of protocols, undertaking research and the review and dissemination of outcomes across the organisation.' Finally, if this is going to be a multicentre trial, think of a clever acronym!

The commonest mistakes people make are to make the trial too complex—attempting to answer too many questions at one time. Very, very few trials ever completely resolve a question, particularly in psychiatry. Deciding what works for whom, how and when, is a long business, in which several trials will contribute to the final answer. Don't over reach yourself. Likewise—keep the basic idea simple. We believe that the aims of any trial should be able to be expressed in a single sentence.

A3 Getting the costs right

Sitting on funding bodies as both authors of this book have done in their time, one of the commonest mistakes made by triallists is to underestimate costs, leading to the embarrassing situation of having to come back with the begging bowl later. In the next section we give a checklist of possible costs. Of course, not all items will be required for all trials, but all require some thought. Listed below are a series of points that may require daily, weekly, monthly or quarterly expenditure. It is essential that these items are budgeted for before the trial begins. Further, it is advisable to have one member of the team responsible for keeping track of what is happening with finances, and reporting to the team about them at regular intervals.

- *The trial co-ordinating staff*: Trial manager (manages the trial), computer programmer, data manager (manages the data), administrator;
- *Sessional input from*: Statistician, health economist, etc.;
- *Consumer input*: Consumer input is becoming increasing important in deciding which questions to ask, and how to ask it. It does not come free—remember to budget for travel, food and so on;
- *Subject allocation to trial*: Randomization system (see Chapter 3);
- *Intervention*: Drug, placebo, packaging, distribution;
- *Measurements*: Questionnaire licensing (if needed);
- *Computing*: Hardware, software, computer consumables;
- *Printing costs*: Questionnaires, protocols, data forms, posters, newsletters;
- *Postage*: Freepost for return of questionnaires, and always budget for multiple mailshots;
- *Telephone/fax/email*: This will be considerable for a multicentre trial;
- *Consumables*: Stationery, telephone, postage, photocopying, freepost licence;
- *Centre costs*: Telephone, photocopying, secretarial/nursing support;
- *Travel*: Site visits, collaborators' meetings;
- *Meeting/travel costs*: Management groups, steering committee and data monitoring committee (obligatory now for all MRC trials).

A4 Collecting and managing the data

The study won't happen unless an intact data set emerges. It is therefore absolutely essential to ensure that data systems are robust and secure. A successful trial will have a well-developed scheme for monitoring the quality of data and for auditing data (see Gassman *et al.*, 1995; George, 1998). Even if the effect of a small number of data errors on scientific conclusions is likely to be small, the effect of discovered errors in the data on public perception and external acceptance of the results can be dramatic. Ensure that all of the points listed below are satisfied before data is entered into any system—remember, *no data—no trial*;

- Is equipment powerful enough for the needs of the trial? Access to a good database management package is often very useful (see Appendix C).
- Are systems protected? Have you complied with the *Data Protection Act*?
- Has the workload been accurately calculated?
- How will data completeness be monitored?
- How will overdue data be monitored?

◆ Will the trial comply with the appropriate regulations? This is a difficult question, since the number of regulations seems to increase from day-to-day. A triallist must be aware of Good Clinical Practice (GP), the entire Research Governance Framework, the European Union Clinical Trials Directive and the similar regulations from the United Kingdom Medicine Controls Agency (MCA) before recruiting a single patient. At the time of writing, all of these are in transition, and it is accurate to say the situation varies from unclear to chaotic. However, in the forthcoming months it is hoped that some order will be restored, not least with the adoption of a uniform Clinical Trials Agreement to be agreed between all NHS Trusts and the pharmaceutical industry, and also with the maturation of the process of Research Governance. The Department of Health website (www.doh.gov.uk) will be a source of updated information as this becomes implemented. Furthermore, assuming that most trials will continue to involve patients of the NHS (at least in the United Kingdom), then your local R&D office will be able to provide the most up-to-date summary of the current regulations.

◆ Test the data system with real data.

◆ Collect data that will give you the outcomes you have specified.

◆ Document the system—if you or your trial co-ordinator is hit by the Number 10 bus, would a stranger be able to recreate the way you have set up and run the trial?

◆ Set up a programme to monitor completeness of data.

◆ Ask your friendly neighbourhood programmer to set up a system to monitor overdue data—has the three-or six-month data been collected on everyone? Some form of prompting system when data becomes overdue could trigger further follow-up efforts.

◆ Build alerts into the data system to warn of potential violations to the protocol.

When it comes to actually collecting the data you will certainly need what is known as a *Case Record Form* (CRF) irrespective of the type of trial you are doing. This will be matched to the requirements of the specific protocol, but will probably need to include sections for each of the following:

◆ Screening form—Baseline data;

◆ Proof of eligibility;

◆ Randomization—allocated study number;

◆ Treatment received (if unblinded);

◆ Follow-up forms—date and method of follow up;

◆ Outcome measures;

◆ Investigations;

◆ Side effects;

◆ Adverse reactions;

- Withdrawal form;
- End of study form.

(It is also essential that this is backed up both in paper form and electronically.)

Investigators need to allow sufficient time for developing and testing CRFs and for receiving and reacting to suggestions from any trial personnel who must use them. Developing the CRF requires people experienced in both form construction and in data collection methods in clinical trials; some useful references are Wright and Haybittle (1979a, b, c) and Barker (1980). The CRFs may be designed to be completed by clinical staff or by patients themselves, although in most clinical trials, particularly in psychiatry, the forms are more likely to be completed by appropriate trial personnel. The study database will include all the data on the CRFs used in the trial as well as possibly data from laboratory tests, etc.

As data collection proceeds it is important to have procedures for monitoring the data. Nowadays many trials have a Data Monitoring Committee (DMC)—sometimes also called a Data Monitoring Ethics Committee (DMEC), whose function is to do what it says 'on the tin'—i.e. to monitor the data from the trial, and advise the Trial Steering Committee appopriately. It decides issues such as the need for interim analyses, and reviews the results of such analyses, including unblinded data if considered necessary. The first role is to monitor trial safety, and to advise when or if trials should be discontinued. Thus the DMC has primarily a responsibility for ethics and safety. Another function, rarely exercised in psychiatric trials, is to conduct interim analyses, and to advise from the unblinded data when the outcome of the trial is already clear, rendering the rest of the study unnecessary. In practice as we discussed earlier, very few psychiatric trials will require interim analyses—most remain underpowered even when completed, and the likelihood of reaching a conclusion earlier than expected is rare indeed. Two additional points are necessary. First, interim analyses must be decided in advance. It is completely wrong to simply 'have a look and see'. Second, membership of the committee must be completely independent of the trial. The trial statistician may however be required to attend to present data and analyses.

A5 Writing the patient information sheet

Always write this in English, not scientific speak. It is always helpful to get a lay-person to check it, and to use your consumer representatives as well. The information sheet should contain the following headings:

- Study title;
- Invitation paragraph;
- What is the study about?
- Why have I been approached?
- Do I have to take part (the answer clearly being no!)?
- What will happen to me if I do take part?
- What do I have to do?

- What is being tested?
- What are the possible side effects of taking part?
- What are the benefits of taking part?
- What are the possible risks or disadvantages of taking part?
- What happens when the trial is over?
- What happens if something goes wrong?
- Is this confidential?
- What will happen to the results of the research?
- Who has funded the study?
- Where can I get further information?

A6 Getting informed consent

Informed consent (IC) should be seen as a process, not merely a signature on a piece of paper. It is a document that is used to prove that the IC process has taken place and that the patient willingly agrees to participate in the study. The new doctrines of Research Governance and the EU Trials Directive mean that all triallists need to be extremely careful that IC is obtained appropriately, and is seen (i.e. documented) to be obtained appropriately.

First, who is going to obtain consent? It must be someone who is qualified, trained and informed to do so. In addition to fulfilling the inclusion criteria, each potential subject's circumstances must be assessed to confirm competency/understand and the support/availability of relatives/carers from the start of the process. EU regulations set out specific criteria that must be met before subjects are entered into trials and more stringent criteria that would apply in the case of minors and adults incapable of giving IC. Further, clinical trials on minors can only be carried out with permission of parents or legal representatives. Trials on adults incapable of giving IC must be sanctioned by a legal representative working for the patient, i.e. a person who can provide independent representation of the patient's interests. However, do remember that patients with mental health problems are not treated any differently from those with physical health problems—what is needed is capacity, which is not normally impaired in either physical or mental disorder, but may be impaired in either. There are no special barriers to obtaining IC from mentally ill patients provided they possess capacity (which basically means the ability to understand the principles of what the trial involves).

It is essential that the patient makes up his/her own mind about participation in the trial, and is enabled to do this through the provision of appropriate information and, particularly in mental health trials, thorough discussion with a relative and/or carer is often necessary.

Many ethics committees are now insisting that there is a time delay between giving information about the trial and obtaining consent. The EU Clinical Trials Directive refers to ' . . . consent being given after a previous meeting where information has been given', suggesting that a potential participant should be given time to think about his/her participation. Unfortunately experience suggests that this will inevitably create further difficulties in trial recruitment, which is already difficult enough. We considered in more detail the meaning of IC in Chapter 2.

A7 Maintaining recruitment

Recruitment is never as good as you think. Like a good marriage, it needs constant work. Here are some tips both when recruiting participants for the trial and in keeping them in the trial:

- Circulate regular newsletters with updates on progress.
- Use posters or letters of congratulation to acknowledge good progress.
- Consider offering incentives for achieving targets, such as T-shirts, mugs or pens, etc. make sure these go to the people doing the work.
- Do you need another collaborator meeting?
- Use opportunities to 'piggy-back' small meetings onto national or international conferences. Organize a session at the next college meeting.
- For multicentre trials, be prepared to visit and revisit any centre that is in danger of failing.
- Liaise with User/Consumer Groups.

A8 Doing the follow-up

Follow-up is a vital part of most clinical trials. Although in Chapter 5 we describe various methods of dealing with missing data, there is no doubt the best method is to avoid the problem as far as possible.

The first point is to think about follow-up before you have started the trial. Hence obtaining consent for follow-up must be part of the initial consent form, since without it you may encounter difficulties in, for example, obtaining change of address data from the patient's general practitioner.

The next point is how are you going to get the information you need. There have been many randomized trials that compare different methods of obtaining responses from postal questionnaires (Edwards *et al.*, 2002). The following have all been shown to significantly increase response rates:

- Monetary incentives;
- Incentives not conditional on responses;
- Short questionnaires;
- Personalized questionnaires and letters;
- Coloured ink;
- Recorded delivery;
- Stamped addressed envelopes;
- First class post;

* Contacting participants before sending questionnaires;
* Reminders;
* Using universities rather than commercial organizations.

A9   Useful web sites

* **British Medical Journal**. http://www.bmj.com. Fully searchable, free electronic library of all BMJ publications, including particular series on statistical issues in the conduct of clinical trials.

* **Central Office for Research Ethics Committees**. http://www.corec.org.uk Up-to-date information on the ever changing rules and regulations governing ethic committees in the National Health Service in the UK.

* **Centre for Evidenced Based Medicine**. http://cebm.jr2.ox.ac.uk Particularly strong on teaching evidence-based medicine and the evidence-based medicine toolkit.

* **Clinical Trial Managers Association** (CTMA). http://www.ctma.org.uk You need to subscribe, but well worth it if you are running a clinical trial.

* **Community of Science Research Funding Database**. http://cos.com. The CONSORT Statement can be found at: http://consort-statement.org. A template trial flow chart is found at aT.

* **The Cochrane Library**. Gives access to the systematic reviews that are produced by the Cochrane collaboration. The abstracts are available free. A subscription fee is charged for full text access. http://www.update-software.com/cochrane

* **Declaration of Helsinki**. http://www.faseb.org/arvo/helsinki.htm

* **Department of Health**. http://www.doh.gov.uk

* **Good Clinical Practice (GCP) Guidelines**. http://www.ich.org/pdfICH/e6.pdf

* **Health Services Research Collaboration**. http://www.epi.bris.ac.uk/hsrc/

* **Institute of Clinical Research**. http://www.acrpi.com. This is a leading clinical research organization. Supplies useful information for industry sponsored trials, trial pharmacists and Good Clinical Practice.

* **ICH Homepage**. http://www.ich.org which contains Good Clinical Practice (GCP) Guidelines.

* **Medical Research Council**. http://www.mrc.ac.uk. Has a wealth of vital information, including MRC Guidelines for Good Clinical Practice in Clinical Trials: MRC Framework for RCTs in Complex Interventions (see Chapter 4): MRC Guidelines on the Ethical Conduct of Research in the Mentally Incapacitated.

* **MRC Trial Managers Network**. http://www.opi.bris.ac.uk/tmn downloadable copy of the MRC Trial Managers Guide, which contains much practical information.

* **Medicines Control Agency**. http://www.mca.gov.uk

- **NHS R&D Health Technology Assessment Programme (HTA)**. http://www.ncchta.org

- **Nuffield Foundation**. http://nuffieldfoundation.org

- **Register of current controlled trials**. http://www.controlled-trials.com. The *meta* register of controlled trials is a searchable, international database of ongoing randomized controlled trials in all areas of healthcare. You should register your clinical trial here.

- **Research Governance**. www.doh.gov.uk/research/documents/rd3/rgforhsclocalimplplans110303.doc

- **Resource Centre for Randomized Trials (RCRT)**. http://www.rcrt.ox.ac.uk. An outstanding resource centre covering most aspects of designing and undertaking RCTs.

Appendix B

Writing a clinical trial report

B1 Introduction

According to Meinert (1986) any investigator who undertakes a trial has a responsibility to make the results obtained from it available for public scrutiny via a published manuscript as soon after the results have been obtained as possible. The goal in the publication should be to provide a clear, concise and accurate description of both how the trial was organized and designed, and the study results. Such a publication should aim to be transparent to its potential readership thus allowing critical appraisal of the quality of the trial and the validity of its findings and conclusions. Sadly there is considerable evidence that the reports of clinical trials are often deficient in several important areas. Altman *et al.* (2001), for example, reviewed the literature that had critically examined clinical trial reports and found the following:

- Information on whether assessment of outcomes was blinded was reported in only 30% of 67 trial reports in four leading journals in 1979 and 1980 (DerSimonian *et al.*, 1982).

- Only 27% of 45 reports published in 1985 defined a primary end point (Pocock *et al.*, 1987).

- Only 43% of 37 trials with negative findings published in 1990 reported a sample size calculation (Moher *et al.*, 1994).

The worry is that poor reporting of the trial may be associated with poor methodology resulting in biased results. This unfortunate state of affairs screams out for some guidelines for the reporting of clinical trials to be agreed, a point made two decades ago by DerSimonian and colleagues:

> Editors could greatly improve the reporting of clinical trials by providing authors with a list of items that they expected to be strictly reported.

But a further decade passed before two independent groups of interested parties (journal editors, trialists and methodologists) published their thoughts and recommendations on the reporting of trials (Standards for Reporting Trials Group, 1994, Working Group on Recommendations for reporting of Clinical Trials, 1994). Collaboration between the two groups eventually resulted in the development of a common set of recommendations set out as the CONSORT (*Con*solidated *S*tandards *of R*eporting *T*rials) statement (Begg *et al.*, 1996).

The core of the CONSORT statement consists of a flow diagram and a checklist both now modified from the original 1996 versions. The latest checklist and flow diagram are given in Altman *et al.* (2001) and are reproduced here in Table B.1 and Fig. B.1.

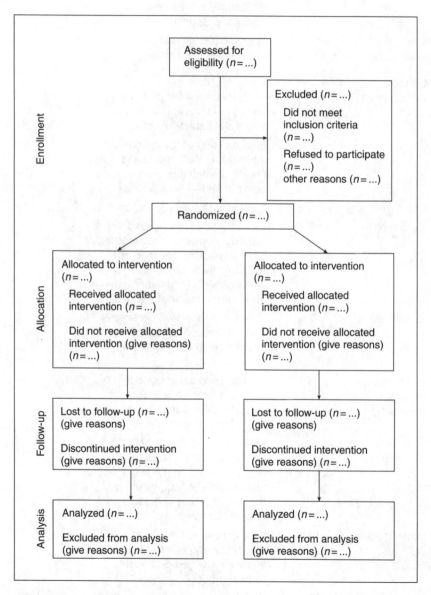

Fig. B.1 CONSORT flowchart.

Table B.1 CONSORT statement checklist.

Paper section and topic	Item number	Descriptor	Reported on page number
Title and abstract	1	How participants were allocated to interventions? (e.g. 'random allocation', 'randomized', or 'randomly assigned')	
Introduction background	2	Scientific background and explanation of rationale.	
Methods			
Participants	3	Eligibility criteria for participants and the settings and locations where the data were collected.	
Interventions	4	Precise details of the interventions intended for each group and how and when they were actually administered.	
Objectives	5	Specific objectives and hypotheses.	
Outcomes	6	Clearly defined primary and secondary outcome measures and, when applicable, any methods used to enhance the quality of measurements (e.g. multiple observations training of assessors).	
Sample size	7	How sample size was determined and, when applicable, explanation of any interim analyses and stopping rules.	
Randomization sequence generation	8	Method used to generate the random allocation sequence, including details of any restriction (e.g. blocking, stratification).	
Allocation concealment	9	Method used to implement the random allocation sequence (e.g. numbered containers or central telephone), clarifying whether the sequence was concealed until interventions were assigned.	
Implementation	10	Who generated the allocation sequence, who enrolled participants, and who assigned participants to their groups?	
Blinding (masking)	11	Whether or not participants, those administering the interventions, and	

| | | those assessing the outcomes were blinded to group assignment. If done, how the success of blinding was evaluated? |
| Statistical methods | 12 | Statistical methods used to compare groups for primary outcome(s); methods for additional analyses, such as and subgroup analyses adjusted analyses. |

Results

Participant flow	13	Flow of participants through each stage (a diagram is strongly recommended). Specifically, for each group report the numbers of participants randomly assigned, receiving intended treatment, completing the study protocol, and analysed for the primary outcome. Describe protocol deviations from study as planned, together with reasons.
Recruitment	14	Dates defining the periods of recruitment and follow-up.
Baseline data	15	Baseline demographic and clinical characteristics of each group.
Numbers analysed	16	Number of participants (denominator) in each group included in each analysis and whether the analysis was by 'intention to treat.' State the results in absolute numbers when feasible (e.g. 10 of 20, not 50%).
Outcomes and estimation	17	For each primary and secondary outcome, a summary of results for each group and the estimated effect size and its precision (e.g. 95% confidence interval).
Ancillary analyses	18	Address multiplicity by reporting any other analyses performed, including subgroup analyses and adjusted analyses, indicating those prescribed and those exploratory.
Adverse events	19	All important adverse events or side effects in each intervention group.

Table B.1 (*continued*)

Paper section and topic	Item number	Descriptor	Reported on page number
Discussion			
Interpretation	20	Interpretation of the results, taking into account study hypotheses, sources of potential bias or imprecision, and the dangers associated with multiplicity of analyses and outcomes.	
Generalizability	21	Generalizability (external validity) of the trial findings.	
Overall evidences	22	General interpretation of the results in the context of current evidence.	

The checklist in Table B.1 identifies 22 items and in which section of the trial report, each should be incorporated. The flow diagram (Fig. B.1) enables reviewers and readers to quickly grasp how many eligible participants were randomly assigned to each arm of the trial. Such information is frequently difficult or impossible to ascertain from trial reports as they are currently presented (Egger *et al.*, 2001, make an attempt to assess the value of flow diagrams in reports of randomized controlled trials, and conclude that such diagrams *are* associated with improved quality, although they suggest that current flow diagram structure is less than ideal and propose a somewhat revised approach).

Altman *et al.* (2001) give a full account of each checklist item and examples of their use; this is essential reading for inexperienced trialists writing their first report and remains an extremely useful *aide memoir* for more experienced investigators. (Further very useful material about writing a clinical trial report is given in Meinert, 1986, Chapter 25; this again has many good examples of good and bad practice.) Here we expand on the material required under a number of the items in Table B.1.

♦ **Title and abstract.** The title and abstract of a clinical trial report are important primarily because they are used in electronic databases that are searched by readers looking for publication of interest. An inappropriate title will often mean, for example, that the paper is overlooked in a systematic review. As Meinert (1986) puts it, 'A good title is neither cute or cryptic.' The title needs to indicate the main topic of the trial in as few words as possible. In reporting RCTs the word randomized is almost *de rigeur*. The accompanying abstract is most useful if it is arranged as a series of headings indicating the design, conduct and analysis of the trial, as well as its conclusion.

♦ **Interventions intended in each group.** Authors need to describe in detail, the study treatments used and how they were administered. This should also include details of the control group intervention. Level of treatment masking and methods of assessing treatment adherence also need to be described.

• **How sample size was determined**. Full details of sample size calculations are needed in clinical trial reports so that readers may, if they wish, replicate the calculations. This requires that the author of the report clearly identifies the primary outcome variable, specifies what was considered a clinically important treatment effect, indicates the statistical test involved, the Type I error rate (significance level) and the power. If the outcome variable is continuous then its assumed variance in the sample size calculation needs to be stated.

• **Statistical methods used to compare groups for primary outcomes**. Authors of clinical trial reports need to make clear the methods of statistical analysis used in the trial. This will enable readers to make a judgement as to whether the methods were appropriate for the type of design used, for the type of outcome measure, etc. Confidence intervals for treatment effects are essential; P-values are of secondary interest only.

Although adequate reporting does not guarantee an adequately designed and analysed trial, the CONSORT statement has, undoubtedly, made a valuable contribution to improving the standard of reporting of clinical trials. (The statement is supported by an increasing number of journals.) But like any such document that attempts to be prescriptive, the entire contents will not find support from every clinical trial investigator, clinician, and statistician. For example, many statisticians will be sorry that the CONSORT statement does not take a strong line *against* the use of P-values rather than simply suggesting that actual P-values ($P = 0.023$, for example) are to be preferred to imprecise threshold reports ($P < 0.001$). Clinical significance cannot be expressed in terms of significance levels, only in terms of the magnitude and direction of treatment effects or differences. Consequently clinical trial reports *must*, in our view at least, report the size of treatment effects and the precision with which they are estimated. As Oakes (1986) rightly comments:

> The significance test relates to what a population parameter is *not*; the confidence interval gives a plausible range for what the parameter *is*.

Appendix C

Useful software for clinical trials

C1 Introduction

Clinical trial investigators may need access to statistical software in both the design and analysis phases of the trial. In this appendix we list details of packages that, in our experience, are most suitable for specific tasks. The list of software is, however, not intended to be comprehensive and there are no doubt many other packages that would provide similar facilities.

C2 Data management

Most statisticians manage data in their statistics package of choice be it, for example, SAS, SPSS, or STATA (see below). Many health professionals keep data in spreadsheets like Microsoft's Excel. In choosing and buying more specialized database software the most important criterion to consider is the capability required of the database. Some useful web sites that can help in making the right choice for a particular trial are:

http://www.symetric.ca

http://www.infogoal.com/dmc/dmcdwh.htm

http:/www-3.ibm.com/software/data

C3 Design

1. *Software for sample size determination*

+ **nQuery Advisor Version 5**. A package for calculating sample size for many types of design and response variable. Available from Statistical Solutions Ltd, 8 South Bank, Crosse's Green, Cork, Ireland. http://www.statsol.ie

- **PASS 2002.** Performs power analysis and calculates sample size. NCSS Statistical Software, 329 North 1000 East, Kaysville, Utah 84037. http://www.ncss.com

2. Software for interim analysis

- **EaSt 2000.** A package for calculating the critical values for various types of interim analysis. Available from Cytel Software Corporation, 675 Massachusetts Avenue, Cambridge, MA 02139, USA. http://www.cytel.com/new.pages/EAST.2.html

- **PEST3.** A package for the planning and evaluation of sequential trials. Available from MPS Research Unit, University of Reading, Earley Gate, Reading RG6 6FN, UK.

C4 Analysis

The most commonly used packages for statistical analysis are:

- **SAS.** SAS Institute Inc, 100 SAS Campus Drive, Cary, NC 27513-2414 USA. http://www.sas.com

- **SPSS.** SPSS Inc, 233 S. Wacker Drive, 11th Floor, Chicago, IL, 60606, USA. http://www.spss.com/

- **STATA.** Stata Corp., 4905 Lakeway Drive, College Station TX 77845, USA. http://www.stata.com

- **S-PLUS.** Insightful Corporation, Global Headquarters, 1700 Westlake Avenue North, Suite 500, Seattle, WA 98109–3044, USA. http://www.insightful.com/

Specialized software for handling missing values includes:

- **SOLAS.** A package for both single and multiple imputation. Available from Statistical Solutions Ltd, 8 South Bank, Crosse's Green, Cork, Ireland. http://www.statsol.ie/solas/solas.htm

- **SAS.** Use proc mi for multiple imputation and proc mianalyze for combining results.

- **S-PLUS.** A comprehensive missing data library is available in S-PLUS 6. Use library(missing).

Software for analysing data in which the dropouts may be informative (see Chapter 5) includes:

- **OSWALD.** A package for dealing with dropouts. Available from Department of Mathematics and Statistics, Fylde College, Lancaster University, Lancaster, LA1 4YF, England. http://www.maths.lancs.ac.uk/Software/Oswald/

- **GLLAMM.** A comprehensive STATA based package that allows a range of models to be fitted to longitudinal data in which dropouts occur. Described in Technical Report 2001/01 Department of Biostatistics and Computing,

Institute of Psychiatry, King's College, London. The program and manual can be downloaded from http://www.iop.kcl.ac.uk/iop/departments/biocomp/programs/gllamm.html

A comprehensive meta-analysis package is available from Biostat Inc., 14, North Dean Street, Englewood, NJ 07631, USA. http://www.metaanalysis.com

References

Abrams DI, Goldman AI, Launer C, Korvick JA, Neaton JD, Crane LR, Grodesky M, Wakefield S, Muth K, Kornegay S, Cohn DL, Harris A, Luskin-Hawk R, Markowitz N, Sampson JH, Thompson M and Deyton L (1994). A comparative trial of didamozine or zalcitaline after treatment with zidovidine in patients with human immunodeficiency virus-infection. *New England Journal of Medicine*, 330, 657–62.

Adams C (1998). Content and quality of 2000 controlled trials in schizophrenia over 50 years. *British Medical Journal*, 317, 1181–4.

Adams C (2002). Randomized controlled trials in schizophrenia: a critical perspective on the literature. *Acta Psychiatrica Scandinavica*, 105, 243–51.

Alexander F and Selesnick ST (1967). *The History of Psychiatry*, New York Harper and Row.

Altman DG (1991). *Practical Statistics for Medical Research*. London: CRC/Chapman and Hall.

Altman D, Schulz K, Moher D, Egger M, Davidoff F, Elbourne D, Gøtzsche PC and Lang T, (2001). The revised CONSORT statement for reporting randomised controlled trials. *Annals of Internal Medicine*, 134, 663–94.

Anscombe FJ (1954). Fixed-sample size analysis of sequential observations. *Biometrics*, 10:89–100.

Antman E, Lau J, Kupelnick B, Mosteller F and Chalmers TC (1992). A comparison of results of meta-analyses of randomized controlled trials and the recommendations of clinical experts. *Journal of the American Medical Association*, 268, 240–8.

Armitage P, McPherson CK and Rowe BC (1969). Repeated significance tests on accumulating data. *Journal of the Royal Statistical Society, Series A*, 132:235–44.

Assmann SF, Pocock SJ, Enos LE and Kasten LE (2000). Subgroup analysis and other (mis) use of baseline data in clinical trials. *Lancet*, 355, 1064–9.

Association AP (2000). *Handbook of Psychiatric Measures*. Washington, DC: American Psychiatric Association.

Anon (2000). A framework for development and evaluation of RCTs for complex interventions to improve health. London: Medical Research Council.

Bailey KR (1987). Inter-study differences: how should they influence the interpretation and analysis of results? *Statistics in Medicine*, 6:351–8.

Barbui C and Hotopf M (2001). Forty years of antidepressant drug trials. *Acta Psychiatrica Scandinavica*, 103, 1–4.

Barrowclough CHG, Tarrier N, Lewis SW, Moring J, O'Brien R, Schofield N and McGovern J (2001). Randomized controlled trial of motivational interviewing, cognitive behavior therapy, and family intervention for patients with comorbid schizophrenia and substance use disorder. *American Journal of Psychiatry*, 158, 1706–13.

Barton S (2000). Which clinical studies provide the best evidence: the best RCT still trumps the best observational study. *British Medical Journal*, 321, 255–6.

Basoğlu M, Marks I, Livanou M and Swinson R (1997). Double blindness procedures, rater blindness and ratings of outcome–observations from a controlled trial, *Archives of General Psychiatry*, 54, 744–8.

Batt JC (1943). One hundred depressive psychoses treated with electrically induced convulsions. *Journal of Mental Science*, 89, 289–96.

Beck AT, Steer A, and Brown GK (1996). *Beck Depression Inventory Manual*, (2nd edn) San Antonia: The Psychological Corporation.

Bennewith O, Stocks N, Gunnell D, Peters TJ, Evans MO and Sharp DJ (2002). General practice based intervention to prevent repeat episodes of deliberate self harm: cluster randomised controlled trial. *British Medical Journal*, 324, 1254–7.

Benson K and Hartz A (2000). A comparison of observational studies and randomized controlled trials. *New England Journal of Medicine*, 342, 1878–86.

Berry DA (1990). Basic principles in designing and analyzing clinical studies In: DA Berry (ed.) *Statistical Methodology in the Pharmaceutical Sciences*. New York: Marcel Dekker, 1–55.

Berry DA (1993). A case for Bayesianism in clinical trials. *Statistics in Medicine*, 12, 1377–93.

Blair RC, Troendle JF and Beck RW (1996). Control of familywise errors in multiple endpoint assessments via stepwise permutation tests. *Statistics in Medicine*, 15, 1107–21.

Bland M (2000). *An Introduction to Medical Statistics*, (3rd edn) Oxford: Oxford University Press.

Bondareff W, Alpert M, Friedhoff AJ, Richter EM, Clary CM and Batzar E (2000). Comparison of sertraline and nerdrophyline in the treatment of major depressive disorder in late life. *American Journal of Psychiatry*, 157, 5, 729–36.

Bradford Hill A (1965). The environment and disease: association or causation?, *Proceedings of the Royal Society of Medicine*, 58, 295–300.

Brewin G and Bradley C (1989). Patient preferences and randomized clinical trials, *British Medical Journal*, 299, 313–15.

Briggs AH and Gray A (1998). The distribution of health care costs and their statistical analysis for economic evaluation. *Journal of Health Service Research and Policy*, 3, 233–45.

Briggs AH, Wonderling DE and Mooney CZ (1997). Pulling cost-effectiveness analysis up by its bootstraps: A non-parametric approach to confidence interval estimation. *Health Economics*, 6, 327–40.

Byar DP (1978). Sound advice for conducting clinical trials. *New England Journal of Medicine*, 297(10), 553–4.

Campbell M, Fitzpatrick R, Haines A, Kinmonth AL, Sandercock P, Spiegelhalter D and Tyrer P (2000). Framework for design and evaluation of complex interventions to improve health. *British Medical Journal*, 321, 694–7.

Carpenter J, Pocock SJ and Lamm CJ (2002). Coping with missing data in clinical trials: a model based approach applied to asthma trials. *Statistics in Medicine*, 21, 1043–66.

Chalmers I (2001). Comparing like with like: some historical milestones in the evolution of methods to create unbiased comparison groups in therapeutic experiments. *International Journal of Epidemiology*, 30, 1156–64.

Chalmers I (2002). MRC Therapeutic Trials Committee's Report on serum treatment of lobar pneumonia, *British Medical Journal*, 1934. In Chalmers I, Milne I, Tröhler U (eds) The James Lind Library.

Chalmers I and Lindley R (2000). Double standards on informed consent to treatment: ignored for a quarter of a century by most professional medical ethicists. In *Informed Consent: Respecting Patients' Rights in Research, Teaching and Practice* (eds L Doyal and J Tobias), London: BMJ Publications, pp. 266–75.

Chalmers TC, Matta R, Smith H and Kunzler A (1977). Evidence favouring the use of anticoagulants in the hospital phase of acute myocardial infarction, *New England Journal of Medicine*, 297, 1091–6.

Chalmers TC and Lau J (1993). Meta-analysis stimulus for change in clinical trials. *Statistical Methods in Medical Research*, 2, 161–72.

Chalmers TC, Celano P, Sacks H and Smith H (1983). Bias in treatment assignment in controlled clinical trials. *New England Journal of Medicine*, 309, 1358–61.

Chuang-Stein C and Tong DM (1997). The impact and implication of regression to the mean on the design and analysis of medical investigations. *Statistical Methods in Medical Search* 6, 115–28.

Concato J, Shah N and Horwitz R (2000). Randomized, controlled trials, observational studies, and the hierarchy of research designs. *New England Journal of Medicine*, 342.

Conley RR and Mahmoud R (2001). A randomized double-blind study of risperidone and olanzapine in the treatment of schizophrenia or schizophrenic disorder. *American Journal of Psychiatry*, 158, 5, 765–74.

Cooper NJ, Sutton AJ and Abrams KR (2002). Decision analytical economics modelling within a Bayesian framework: Application to prophylactic antibiotics use for caesarean section. *Statistical Methods in Medical Research*, 11, 1–22.

Copas JB and Shi JQ (2001). A sensitivity analysis for publication bias in systematic reviews. *Statistical Methods in Medical Research*, 10, 251–66.

Cornfield J (1976). Recent methodological contributions to clinical trials. *American Journal of Epidemiology*, 104, 408–21.

Cotton HA (1922). The etiology and treatment of the so called functional psychoses. *American Journal of Psychiatry*, 2, 157–210.

Cox DR (1998). Discussion. *Statistics in Medicine*, 17, 387–9.

Cramer JA, Collins JF and Mallson RH (1988). Can categorization of patient background problems be used to determine early termination in a clinical trial? *Contr. Clin. Trials*, 9, 47–63.

Crawford MJ, W T, Rutter D, Sensky T and Tyrer P (2002). Evaluating new treatments in psychiatry: the potential value of combining qualitative and quantitative research methods. *International Review Of Psychiatry*, 14, 6–11.

Davies D and M Shepherd (1955). Reserpine in the treatment of anxious patients. *Lancet*, i: 117–20.

De Mets DL (1987). Methods for combining randomized clinical trials: strengths and limitations. *Statistics in Medicine*, 6, 341–8.

Deale A, Chalder T, Marks IM and Wessely S (1997). Cognitive behaviour therapy for chronic fatigue syndrome. A randomized controlled trial. *American Journal of Psychiatry*, 154, 408–14.

Dennis MOS, Slattery J, Staniforth T and Warlow C (1997). Evaluation of a stroke family care worker: Results of a randomised controlled trial. *British Medical Journal*, 314, 1071–6.

Dennis M (1997). Why we didn't ask patients for their consent: Commentary. *British Medical Journal*, 314, 1077.

Der Simonian R and Laird N (1986). Meta-analysis in clinical trials. *Controlled Clinical Trials*, 7, 177–88.

Diggle PJ and Kenward MG (1994). Informative drop-out in longitudinal analysis (with discussion). *Applied Statistics*, 43, 49–93.

Diggle PJ (1988). An approach to the analysis of repeated measures. *Biometrics*, 44, 959–71.

Diggle PJ (1998). Dealing with missing values in longitudinal studies, In: B. S. Everitt and G. Dunn (eds). *Statistical Analysis of Medical Data: New Developments*. London: Arnold, 203–28.

Diggle PJ, Liang KY and Zeger SL (1994). *Analysis of Longitudinal Data*. Oxford: Oxford Scientific Publications.

Doll R (1998). Controlled trials: the 1948 watershed. *British Medical Journal*, 317, 1217–20.

Donner A and Klar NS (2000). *Design and Analysis of Cluster Randomization Trials in Health Research.* London: Arnold.

Dunn, G (1996). Statistical methods for measuring outcomes. In *Mental Health Outcome Measures* G Thornicroft and M Tansella (eds), Berlin: Springer Verlag, pp. 3–13.

Dunn G, Maracy M, Dowrick C, Ayuso-Mateos JL, Dalgard OS, Page H, Lehtinen V, Cassey P, Wilkinson C, Vázquez-Barquero JL and Wilkinson G (2003). Estimating psychological treatment effects from an RCT with both non-compliance and loss to follow-up: the ODIN trial, *British Journal of Psychiatry,* In press.

Duval S and Tweedie RL (2000). A nonparametric 'trim and fill' method of accounting for publication bias in meta-analysis. *Journal of the American Statistical Association,* 95, 89–98.

Easterbrook PJ, Berlin JA, Gepalas R and Mathews DR (1991). Publication bias in research. *Lancet,* 337, 867–72.

Ederer F (1998). *History of clinical trials,* In Encyclopedia of Biostatistics Vol 3, P Armitage and T Colton (eds), Wiley, Chichester.

Efron B and Feldman D (1991). Compliance as an explanatory variable in clinical trials. *Journal of the American Statistical Association,* 86, 9–17.

Efron B (1998). Foreword in special issue on Analyzing Non-Compliance in Clinical Trials. *Statistics in Medicine,* 17, 249–50.

Ekles J and Elkes C (1954). Effect of chlorpromazine on the behaviour of chronically over-active psychotic patients. *British Medical Journal* i, 560–5.

Ellenberg SS, Fleming TR and De Mets DL (2002). *Data Monitoring Committees in Clinical Trials: A Practical Perspective.* Chichester: Wiley.

Ellwood P (1988). Outcomes management: a technology of patient experience. *New England Journal of Medicine,* 318, 1549–6.

Everitt BS and Pickles A (2000). *Statistical Aspects of the Design and Analysis of Clinical Trials.* London: Imperial College Press.

Everitt BS (2002a). *Modern Medical Statistics.* London: Arnold.

Everitt BS (2002b). *The Cambridge Dictionary of Statistics,* (2nd ed) Cambridge: Cambridge University Press.

Eysenck H (1978). An exercise in mega silliness. *American Psychologist,* 33, 517.

Farmer A, McGuffin P and Williams J (2002). *Measuring Psychopathology.* Oxford, Oxford University Press.

Featherstone K and Donovan J (2002). 'Why don't they just tell me straight, why allocate it?' The struggle to make sense of participating in a randomised controlled trial. *Social Science and Medicine,* 55, 709–19.

Feinstein AR (1991). Intention-to-treat policy for analyzing randomized trials: Statistical distortions and neglected clinical challenges, Chapter 28 In: J A Cramer and B Spilker, (eds) *Patient Compliance in Medical Practice and Clinical Trials.* New York: Raven Press Ltd.

Fitzgerald OWS (1943). Experiences in the treatment of depressive stats by electrically induced convulsions. *Journal of Mental Science,* 89, 73–80.

Fleiss JL (1993). The statistical basis of meta-analysis. *Statistical Methods in Medical Research,* 2, 121–45.

Fleiss JL (1986). *The Design and Analysis of Clinical Experiments,* Wiley, New York.

Fontanet AL, Saba J, Chandelying V, Sakondhquat C, Bhiruleus P, Chongsomchai C, Lriwat O, Tovanabutra S, Dally L, Lange JM and Rojanapithayakorn W (1998). Protection against sexually transmitted diseases by granting sex workers in Thailand the choice of using the male or female condom: results from a randomized controlled trial. *AIDS,* 12, 1851–9.

Foucault M (1961). *Madness and Civilization: a history of insanity in the Age of Reason,* translated from the French by Richard Howard, Tavistock London 1967. (Originally published in French as *Histoire de la Folie.*)

Friedman LM, Furberg CD and De Mets DL (1985). *Fundamentals of Clinical Trials,* (2nd edn) Littleton, MA: PSB Publishing.

Freiman JA, Chalmers TC and Smith H (1978). The importance of beta, the type II error and sample size in the design and interpretation of the randomized control trial: surgery of 'negative' trials. *New England Journal of Medicine,* 299, 690–4.

Frison L and Pocock SJ (1992). Repeated measures in clinical trials: analysis using mean summary statistics and its implications for design. *Statistics in Medicine,* 11, 1685–1704.

Gardner MJ and Altman DG (1986). Confidence intervals rather than p-values: estimation rather than hypothesis testing. *British Journal Medicine,* 292, 746.

Geddes J (2002). Can we conduct some large simple trials in bipolar disorder? *Bipolar Disorder,* 4 (suppl 1), 62–3.

Gibbons RD, Hecteker D and Elkin H (1993). Some conceptual and statistical issues in analysis of longitudinal psychiatric data. *Archives of General Psychiatry,* 50, 739–50.

Gilbody S, Wahlbeck K and Adams C (2002). Randomized controlled trials in schizophrenia: a critical perspective on the literature. *Acta Psychiatrica Scandinavica,* 105, 243–51.

Gilbody S (2002). Outcome measurement in psychiatry: a critical review of patient based outcome measurements in psychiatric research and practice. Ph D Thesis: York: York University.

Givens GH, Smith DD and Tweedie RL (1997). Publication bias in meta-analysis: a Bayesian data-augmentation approach to account for issues exemplified in the passive smoking debate (with discussion). *Statistical Science,* 12, 244–5.

Glass G (1976). Primary care, secondary and meta analysis of research. *Education Research,* 5, 3–8.

Glasgow RE, Lichtenstein E, Wilder D, Hall R, McRae SG and Liberty B (1995). The tribal tobacco policy project. Working with North West Indian tribes on smoking policies. *Preventative Medicine,* 24, 434–40.

Glasziou PP and Sanders SL (2002). Investigating causes of heterogeneity in systematic reviews. *Statistics in Medicine,* 21, 1503–12.

Goetghebeur EJT and Shapiro SH (1996). Analyzing non-compliance in clinical trials: Ethical imperative or mission impossible? *Statistics in Medicine,* 15, 2813–26.

Gordon BL (1949). *Medicine Throughout Antiquity.* Philadelphia: Davies.

Gotzsche PC and Lange B (1991). Comparison of search strategies for recalling double-blind trials from MEDLINE. *Danish Medical Bulletin,* 38, 476–8.

Greenwald AG (1975). Consequences of prejudice against the null hypothesis. *Psychological Bulletin,* 85, 845–57.

Group, FISoISC (1995). ISIS-4: a randomised factorial trial assessing early oral captopril, oral mononitrate and intravenous magnesium sulphate in 58,050 patients with suspected acute myocardial infarction. *Lancet,* 345, 669–85.

Grundy CT, Lunnen KM, Lambert MJ, Ashton JE and Tovey DR (1994). The Hamilton Rating Scale for Depression: one scale or many? *Clinical Psychology: Science and Practice,* 1, 197–204.

Guthrie E, Creed R, Davison D and Tamenson B (1993). A randomized controlled trial of psychotherapy in patients with refractory irritable bowel syndrome. *British Journal of Psychology,* 163, 321.

Hamilton M (1969). A rating scale for depression. *Journal of Neurology, Neurosurgery and Psychiatry,* 23, 56–62.

Hartz A (2000). A comparison of observational studies and randomized controlled trials. *New England Journal of Medicine,* 342, 1878–86.

Healy D (1997). *The Antidepressant Era*. Cambridge, Mass., Harvard University Press.

Heinrichs D, Hanlon T and Carpenter W (1984). The Quality of Life Scale: an instrument for rating the schizophrenic deficit syndrome. *Schizophrenia Bulletin*, 10, 388–98.

Heitjan DF (1997). Bayesian interim analysis of phase II cancer clinical trials. *Statistics in Medicine*, 16, 1791–802.

Hill A (1966). Reflections on the controlled trial. *Annals of Rheumatic Diseases*, 25, 107–113.

Hjalmarson A, Elmfeldt D, Herlitz J, Holmberg S, Nyberg G, Ryden L, Swedberg K, Waagstein F, Waldenstrum A, Vedin A, Wedel H, Wilhelmsen L and Wilhelmsen C (1981). A double blind trial of metoprolol in acute myocardial infarction—effects on mortality. *Circulation*, 64, 140.

Hlatky MA, Boothroyd DB and Johnstone IM (2002). Economic evaluation in long-term clinical trials. *Statistics in Medicine*, 21, 2879–88.

Holtzman JL, Kiam DC, Berry DC, Mottonen L, Barret G, Harrison LI and Conrad GJ (1987). The pharmacodynamic and pharmacokinetic interaction of flecouride acetate and propranolol; effects on cardiac function and drug clearance. *European Journal of Clinical Pharmacology*, 33, 97–9.

Hopewell S, Clarke M, Lusher A, Lefebvre C and Westby M (2002). A comparison of hand-searching versus MEDLINE searching to identify reports of randomized controlled trials. *Statistics in Medicine*, 21(11), 1625–34.

Horton R (2001). The clinical trial: deceitful, disputable, unbelievable, unhelpful, and shameful–What next? *Controlled Clinical Trials*, 22, 593–604.

Horwitz R (2000). Randomized, controlled trials, observational studies, and the hierarchy of research designs. *New England Journal of Medicine*, 342.

Hotopf M (2002). The pragmatic randomised controlled trial. *Advances in Psychiatric Treatment*, 8, 326–33.

Hotopf M, Churchill R and Lewis G (1999). Pragmatic randomised controlled trials in psychiatry. *British Journal of Psychiatry*, 175, 217–23.

Hotopf M, Lewis G and Normand C (1997). Putting trials on trial–the costs and consequences of small trials in depression: a systematic review of methodology. *Journal of Epidemiology and Community Health*, 51, 354–8.

Hotopf M and Normand C (1997). Putting trials on trial–the costs and consequences of small trials in depression: a systematic review of methodology. *Journal of Epidemiology and Community Health*, 51, 354–8.

Hrobjartsson AGP (2001). Is the placebo powerless? An analysis of clinical trials comparing placebo with no treatment. *New England Journal of Medicine*, 344, 1594–602.

Hsieh FY (1987). A simple method of sample size calculation for unequal sample-size designs that use the logrank or t-test. *Statistics in Medicine*, 6, 577–81.

Hunt S and McKenna S (1992). A new measure of quality of life in depression: testing the reliability and constructive validity of the QLDS. *Health Policy*, 22, 321–30.

Irwin M, Lovitz A, Marder SR, Mintz J, Winsdale WJ, Van Putten T and Mills MJ (1985). Psychotic patients' understanding of informed consent, *American Journal of Psychiatry*, 142, 1351–4.

Ishak W and Burt T (eds) (2002) *Outcome Measurement in Psychiatry: A Critical Review*. Washington: American Psychiatric Association.

Iyenger SI and Greenhouse JB (1988). Selection models and the file drawer problem. *Statistical Science*, 3, 109–17.

Jennison C and Turnbull B (1989). Interim analysis: The repeated confidence interval approach (with discussion). *Journal of the Royal Statistical Society, Series B*, 51, 305–62.

Johnson T (1998). Clinical trials in psychiatry: Background and statistical perspective. *Statistical Methods in Medical Research*, 7, 209–34.

Joyce J, Rabe Hesketh S and Wessely S (1998). Reviewing the reviews: the example of chronic fatigue syndrome. *Journal of the American Medical Association*, 280, 264–6.

Juni P, Witschi A, Bloch R and Egger M (1999). The hazards of scoring the quality of clinical trials for meta-analysis. *Journal of the American Medical Association*, 282, 1054–60.

Kaptchuk T (1998). Intentional ignorance: A history of blind assessment and placebo controls in medicine. *Bulletin of the History of Medicine*, 72, 389–433.

Karagulla S (1950). Evaluation of electrical convulsion therapy as compared with conservative methods of treatment of depressive states. *Journal of Mental Science*, 96, 1060–91.

Kemp R, Hayward P, Applewhaite G, Everitt B and David A (1996). Compliance therapy in psychotic patients: randomised controlled trial. *British Medical Journal*, 312, 345–9.

Kerr C, Robinson E, Stevens A, Braunholtz D, Edwards S, Lilford R (2004). Randomisation in trials: do potential trial participants understand it and find it helpful? *Journal of Medical Ethics*. In Press.

Kerry S and Bland M (1998). Analysis of a trial randomised in clusters. *British Medical Journal*, 316, 54.

Kessler R and Frank R (1997). The impact of psychiatric disorder on work loss days. *Psychological Medicine*, 27, 861–73.

Kim HL, Streltzer J and Goebert D (1999). St John's Wort for depression: a meta-analysis of well-defined clinical trials, *Journal of Nervous and Mental Disorders*, 187, 532–8.

Kirsch I and Sapirstein G (1998). Listening to Prozac but hearing placebo: A meta-analysis of antidepressant medication. *Prevention and Treatment*, 1, 002A.

Kleijnen J (1997). Current controversies in the application of meta-analysis (with special reference to oncological treatments). A commentary. *Pharmacy World & Science*, 19(3), 117–8.

Kleijnen J, Gotzsche P, Kunz R, Oxman A and Chalmers I (1997). So what's special about randomization? In A. Maynard I. Chalmers Eds. *Non-Random Reflections on Health Services Research*. London: BMJ Publishing Groups.

Kopeloff N and Cheney HG (1923). Focal infection and mental disease. *American Journal of Psychiatry*, 3, 149–98.

Kroenke K, West S, Swindle R, Gilsenan A, Eckert G, Dolor R, Stang P, Zhou X, Hays R and Weinberger M (2001). Similar effectiveness of paroxetine, fluoxetine, and sertraline in primary care: a randomized trial. *Journal of the American Medical Association*, 2947–55.

Kuipers E, Fowler D, Garety P, Chishopin D, Freeman D, Dunn G, Bebbington P and Hadley C (1998). London-East Anglia randomised controlled trial of cognitive-behavioural therapy for psychosis III Follow-up and economic evaluation at 18 months. *British Journal of Psychiatry*, 173, 61–8.

Kunz R and Oxman AD (1998). The unpredictability paradox: review of empirical comparisons of randomized and non-randomised clinical trials, *British Medical Journal*, 317, 1185–90.

Laird NM (1988). Missing data in longitudinal studies. *Statistics in Medicine*, 7, 305–15.

Lan KKG, De Mets DL (1983). Discrete sequential boundaries for clinical trials. *Biometrika*, 70, 659–63.

Lasater TM, Becker DM, Hill MN and Gans KM (1997). Synthesis of findings and issues from religious–based cardiovascular disease prevention trials. *Annals of Epidemiology*, 7, 546–53.

Le Fanu J (1999). *The Rise and Fall of Modern Medicine*. London: Abacus.

Leber P (2000). The use of placebo control groups in the assessment of psychiatric drugs: an historical context. *Biological Psychiatry*, 47, 699–706.

Lee YJ (1983). Quick and simple approximations of sample sizes for comparing two independent binomial distributions: Different sample-size curve. *Biometrics*, 40, 239–42.

Lehmann H (1993). Before they called it Psychopharmacology. Neuropsychopharmacology. *Neuropharmacology*, 8, 291–303.

Leonard CO, Chase GA and Childs B (1972). Genetic Counseling: a consumer's view, *New England Journal of Medicine*, 287, 433–9.

Leese MN, White IR, Schene AH, Koetr MWJ, Ruggeri M, and Gaite L (2001). Reliability in multi-site psychiatric studies. *International Journal of Methods in Psychiatric Research*, 10, 29–41.

Levine RJ and Lebacqz KA (1979). Ethical considerations in clinical trials. *Clinical Pharmacology & Therapeutics*, 25, 728–41.

Lewis AJ (1946). On the place of physical treatment in psychiatry. *British Medical Journal*, 3, 22–4.

Lewis G (1991). Observer Bias and the Assessment of Anxiety and Depression. *Social Psychiatry and Psychiatric Epidemiology*, 26, 265–72.

Liang KY and Zeger SL (1986). Longitudinal data analysis using generalized linear models. *Biometrika*, 73, 13–22.

Lind J (1753). *A Treatise of the Scurvey* reprinted in Lind's Treatise on Scurvey CP Stewart and D Guthrie (eds), Edinburgh University Press, Edinburgh (1953) Sands-Murray-Cochron, Edinburgh.

Linde K, Ramirez G, Mulrow CD, Pauls A, Weidenhammer W and Melchart D (1996). St John's Wort for depression–an overview and meta-analysis of randomized clinical trials, *British Medical Journal*, 313, 253–8.

Little RJA (1995). Modelling the drop-out mechanism in repeated measures studies. *Journal of the American Statistical Association*, 90, 1112–21.

Litz BT, Gray M, Bryant R, *et al.* (2002). Early intervention for trauma: current status and future directions. *Clinical Psychology: Science and Practice*, 9, 112–34.

Lubsen J and Pocock SJ (1994). Factorial trials in cardiology: Pros and Cons. *European Heart Journal*, 15, 585–8.

Marshall M, Lockwood A, Bradley C, Adams C, Joy C and Fenton M (2000). Unpublished rating scales–a major source of bias in randomised controlled trials of treatments for schizophrenia? *British Journal of Psychiatry*, 176, 249–52.

Mason S, Tovey P and Long A (2002). Evaluating complementary medicine: methodological challenges of randomised controlled trials, *British Medical Journal*, 325, 832–4.

Matthews JNS (1994). Discussion of Diggle and Kenward. *Applied Statistics*, 43, 49–93.

Matthews JNS, Altman DG, Campbell MJ and Royston P (1990). Analysis of serial measurements in medical research. *British Medical Journal*, 300, 230–5.

McHugh RB and Lee CT (1984). Confidence estimation and the size of a clinical trial. *Controlled Clinical Trials*, 5, 157–64.

McKee M, Britton A, Black N, McPherson K, Sanderson C and Bain C (1999). Interpreting the evidence: choosing between randomised and non-randomised studies. *British Medical Journal*, 319, 312–15.

McNamara B, Ray JL, Arthurs OJ and Boniface S (2001). Transcranial magnetic stimulation for depression and other psychiatric disorders. *Psychological Medicine*, 31: 1141–6.

McPherson K (1982). On choosing the number of interim analyses in clinical trials. *Statistics in Medicine*, 1, 25–36.

McPherson K, Britton A and Wennberg J (1997). Are randomized controlled trials controlled? Patient preferences and unblind trials. *Journal of the Royal Society of Medicine*, 90, 652–6.

Medical Research Council (1944). Patulin Clinical Trials Committee. Clinical trial of patulin in the common cold. *Lancet*, 2, 373–5.

Medical Research Council (1948). Streptomycin treatment of pulmonary tuberculosis. *British Medical Journal*, ii, 769–82.

Medical Research Council (1965). Clinical Trial of the treatment of depressive illness. *British Medical Journal*, i, 881–6.

Meinert CL (1986). *Clinical Trials–Design, Conduct and Analysis*. New York: Oxford University Press.

Meier P (1987). Commentary. *Statistics in Medicine*, 6, 329–31.

Miller F (2000). Placebo-controlled trials in psychiatric research: an ethical perspective. *Biological Psychiatry*, 47, 707–16.

Moertel CG, Fleming TR, Macdonald JS, Haller DG, Laurie JA, Goodman PJ, Ungerleider JS, Emerson WA, Tormey DC, Glick JH, Veeder MH and Mailliard JA (1990). Levamisole and Fluorairacil for adjustment therapy of resected colon carcinoma. *New England Journal of Medicine*, 332, 353–8.

Moher D, Jeidad AR, Nichol G, *et al.* (1995). Assessing the quality of randomized controlled trials: An annotated bibliography of scales and checklists. *Controlled Clinical Trials*, 16, 62–73.

Muijen M, Marks I and Connolly J (1992). Home based care and standard hospital care for patients with severe mental illness: a randomised controlled trial. *British Medical Journal*, 304, 749–54.

Manning WG and Mullahy J (2001). Estimating log models: to transform or not to transform? *Journal of Health Economics*, 20(4), 461–94.

Mulrow C (1987). The medical review article: state of the art. *Annals of Internal Medicine*. 106, 485–8.

Murray GD and Findlay JG (1998). Correcting for bias caused by dropouts in hypertension trials, *Statistics in Medicine*, 7, 941–6.

Napier FJ (1944). Death from electrical convulsion therapy. *Journal of Mental Science*, 90, 845–78.

Oakes M (1986). *Statistical Inference: A Commentary for the Social and Behavioural Sciences*. Chichester: John Wiley & Sons.

Oakes M (1993). The Logic and role of meta-analysis in clinical research. *Statistical Methods in Medical Research*, 2, 147–60.

O'Brien BJ and Briggs AH (2002). Analysis of uncertainty in health care cost-effectiveness studies: an introduction to statistical issues and methods. *Statistical Methods in Medical Research*, 11, 1–14.

O'Brien PC (1984). Procedures for comparing samples with multiple end points. *Biometrics*, 40, 1079–87.

O'Brien PC and Fleming TR (1979). A multiple testing procedure for clinical trials. *Biometrics*, 35, 549–56.

O'Hagan A and Stevens JW (2002). Bayesian methods for design and analysis of cost-effectiveness trials in evaluation of health care technologies. *Statistical Methods in Medical Research*, 11, 1–22.

Oldham PD (1962). A note on the analysis of repeated measurements of the same subjects. *Journal Chronic Disease*, 15, 969–77.

Owley T, McMahon W, Cook EH, Laulhere T, South M, Zellmer M, Shernoff ES, Lainhart J, Modahl CB, Corsello C, Ozonoff S, Risi S, Lord C, Leventhal BL and Filipek PA (2001). Multisite, double-blind, placebo-controlled trial of porcine secretin in autism. *Journal of the American Academy of Child and Adolescent Psychiatry*, 40, 1293–99.

Palmer CR (2002). Ethics, data-dependent designs and the strategy of clinical trials: time to start learning-as-we-go? *Statistical Methods in Medical Research*, 11, 381–402.

Pampallona S and Tsiatis AA (1994). Group sequential designs for one-sided and two-sided hypothesis testing with provision for early stopping in favour of the null hypothesis. *Journal of Statistical Planning and Inference*; 42:19–35.

Patrick D and Erickson P (1993). *Health Studies and Health Policy*. New York: Oxford University Press.

Peduzzi P, Wittes J and Detre K (1993). Analysis-as-randomized and the problem of non-adherence–an example from the veterans affairs randomized trial of coronary-artery bypass surgery. *Statistics in Medicine*, 12, 1185–95.

Persons J and Silberschatz G (1998). Are results of randomized controlled trials useful to psychotherapists? *Journal of Consulting and Clinical Psychology*, 66, 126–35.

Peto R, Pike MC and Armitage P (1976). Design and analysis of randomized clinical trials requiring prolonged observation of each patient: I Introduction and Design. *British Journal of Cancer*, 34, 585–612.

Peveler R, George C, Kinmonth A, Campbell M and Thompson C (1999). Effect of anti-depressant drug counselling and information leaflets on adherence to drug treatment in primary care: randomised controlled trial. *British Medical Journal*, 319, 612–15.

Piaggio GCG, Villar J, Pinol A, Bakketeig L, Lumbiganon P, Bergsjo P, Al-Mazrou Y, Ba'aqeel, H, Belizan, JM, Farnot U and Berendes H (2001). Methodological considerations on the design and analysis of an equivalence stratified cluster randomization trial. *Statistics in Medicine*, 20, 401–16.

Piantadosi S (1997) Clinical Trials: *A Methodological Perspective*, New york: Wiley.

Pickering GW (1949). The place of the experimental method in medicine. *Proceedings of the Royal Society of Medicine*, 42, 229–34.

Pinheiro JC and Bates DM (2001). *Mixed Effects Models in S and S-PLUS*. New York: Springer.

Pinheiro JC and De Mets DL (1997). Estimating and reducing bias in group sequential designs with Gaussian independent increment structure. *Biometrika*, 84, 831–45.

Robinson E, Kerr C, Edwards S, Stevens A, Braunholtz D, Lilford R (2004). Lay conceptions of the ethical and scientific justification for randomisation in clinical trials. *Social Science in Medicine*. In Press.

Rosner G and Tsiatis AA (1989). The impact that group sequential tests would have made on ECOG clinical trials. *Statistics in Medicine*, 8, 505–16.

Rothman K and Michels K (1994). The continuing unethical use of placebo controls. *New England Journal of Medicine*, 331, 394–8.

Rothwell P (1995). Can overall results of clinical trials be applied to all Patients? *Lancet*, 345, 1616–19.

Rubin DB (1976). Inference and Missing Data. *Biometrika*, 63, 581–92.

Russell D (1996). *Scenes from Bedlam: A History of the Bethlem Royal and Maudsley Hospitals*. Scutari Press.

Sackett DL, Rosenberg WMC, Gray JAM and Richardson WS (1996). Evidence based medicine: what it is and what it isn't. *British Medical Journal*, 312, 71–2.

Sacks H, Berrier J, Reitman D, *et al.* (1987). Meta-analyses of randomized controlled trials. *New England Journal of Medicine*, 316, 450–5.

Sacks H, Chalmers T and Smith H (1982). Randomized versus historical controls for clinical trials. *American Journal of Medicine*, 72, 233–40.

Sacks HS, Chalmers TC, Blum AL, Berrier J and Pagano D (1990). Endoscopic homeostasis: An effective therapy for bleeding peptic ulcers. *Journal of the American Medical Association*, 264, 494–9.

Sargent W and Slater E (1944). An *Introduction to Physical Methods of Treatment in Psychiatry*. Edinburgh: Livingstone.

Schafer JL (1999). Multiple imputation: A Primer. *Statistical Methods in Medical Research*, 8, 3–16.

Schellings RKA, ter Riet G and Sturmans F (1999). The Zelen design may be the best choice for a heroin-provision experiment. *Journal of Clinical Epidemiology*, 52, 503–7.

Schoenfield DA (1983). Sample size formula for the proportional hazards regression model. *Biometrika*, 39, 499–503.

Schou M, J-Neilsen N, Stromgren E and Voldby H (1954). The treatment of manic-psychoses by the administration of lithium salts. *Journal Neurological Psychiatry*, 17, 250–60.

Schultz K and Grimes D (2002). Allocation concealment in randomised trials: defending against deciphering. *Lancet*, 359, 614–18.

Schultz K, Chalmers I, Grimes D and Altman DG (1994). Assessing the quality of randomization from reports of controlled trials published in obstetrics and gynecology journals. *Journal of the American Medical Association*, 272, 125–8.

Schultz K, Chalmers I, Hayes R and Altman DG (1995). Empirical evidence of bias: dimensions of methodological quality associated with estimates of treatments effects in controlled trials. *Journal of the American Medical Association*, 273, 408–12.

Schwartz D and Lellouch J (1967). Explanatory and pragmatic attitudes in therapeutic trials, *Journal of Chronic Disorders*, 20, 637–48.

Scott NW, McPherson GC, Ramsay CR and Campbell MK (2002). The method of minimization for allocation to clinical trials: a review. *Controlled Clinical Trials*, 23, 662–74.

Senn S (1994a). Repeated measures in clinical trials: analysis using mean summary statistics and its implications for design. *Statistics in Medicine*, 13, 197–8.

Senn S (1994b). Testing for baseline balance in clinical trials. *Statistics in Medicine*, 13, 1715–26.

Senn S (1997). *Statistical Issues in Drug Development*. Chichester: John Wiley & Sons.

Senn S (1998). Some controversies in planning and analysing multi-centre trials. *Statistics in Medicine*, 17, 1753–65.

Senn S (2001). *Cross-over Trials*, (2nd ed). Chichester: Wiley.

Sensky T, Turkington D, Kingdon D, Scott JL, Scott J, Siddle R, O'Carroll M and Barnes TR (2000). A randomized controlled trial of cognitive-behavioral therapy for persistent symptoms in schizophrenia resistant to medication. *Archives of General Psychiatry*, 57, 165–72.

Shelton RC, Gelenberg A, Dunner DL, Hirschfeld R, Thase ME, Rydiard RD, Crits-Cristoph P, Gallop R, Todd L, Heller stein D, Goodnick P, Keitner G, Stahl SM, Halbreich U (2001). Effectiveness of St John's Wort in major depression – A randomized controlled trial, *Journal of the American Medical Association*, 285, 1978–86.

Shepherd M (1959). Evaluation of drugs in the treatment of depression. *Canadian Psychiatric Association Journal*, 4: 120–8.

Sibbald B and Roland M (1998). Why are randomised controlled trials important? *British Medical Journal*, 316, 201.

Silberschatz G (1998). Are results of randomized controlled trials useful to psychotherapists? *Journal of Consulting and Clinical Psychology*, 66, 126–35.

Silliman NP (1997a). Nonparametric classes of weight functions to model publication bias. *Biometrika*, 84, 909–18.

Silliman NP (1997b). Hierarchical selection models with applications in meta analysis. *Journal of the American Statistical Association*, 92, 926–36.

Silverman WA (1985). *Human Experimentation: A Guided Step into the Unknown*. Oxford: Oxford Medical Publications.

Simon G, Vonkorff M and Barlow W (1995). Health care costs of primary care patients with recognized depression. *Archives of General Psychiatry*, 52, 850–6.

Simon R (1991). A decade of progress in statistical methodology for clinical trials. *Statistics in Medicine*, 10, 1789–1817.

Simon R (1994). Some practical aspects of the interim monitoring of clinical trials. *Statistics in Medicine*, 13, 1401–9.

Slade M and Priebe S (2001). Are randomised controlled trials the only gold that glitters? *British Journal of Psychiatry*, 179, 286–7.

Slade M (2002). What outcomes to measure in routine mental health services, and how to assess them: a systematic review. *Australian and New Zealand Journal of Psychiatry*, 36, 743–53.

Slade M, Kuipers M and Priebe S (2002). Mental health services research methodology. *International Review of Psychiatry*, 14, 12–18.

Smith H (1982). Randomized versus historical controls for clinical trials. *American Journal of Medicine*, 72, 233–40.

Smith ML (1980). Publication bias and meta-analysis. *Evaluating Education*, 4, 22–4.

Smith R (1997). Informed consent: The intricacies–Should the BMJ reject all studies that do not include informed consent? *British Medical Journal*, 314, 1059–60.

Smithells R (1975). Iatrogenic hazards and their effects. *Postgraduate Medical Journal*, 51, 39–52.

Snaith R (1996). Present use of the Hamilton Depression Rating Scale: Observations on method of assessmnet in research of depressive disorders. *British Journal of Psychiatry*, 168, 594–7.

Sommer A, Tarwotjo I, Djunaedi E, West KP, Loeden AA and Tilden R (1986). Impact of vitamin A supplementation on childhood mortality. *Lancet*, 1, 1169–73.

Souhami RL (1994). The clinical importance of early stopping of randomized trials in cancer treatments. *Statistics in Medicine*, 13, 1293–5.

Spiegelhalter DJ, Freedman LS and Parmar MKB (1994). Bayesian approaches to randomized trials. *Journal of the Royal Statistical Society, Series A*, 157, 357–416.

Spilker B (1991). *Guide to Clinical Trials*, Wiley, New York.

Sterlin TD (1959). Publication decisions and their possible effects on inferences drawn from tests of significance–or vice versa. *Journal of the American Statistical Association*, 54, 30–4.

Swartz MSSJ, Hiday VA, Wagner HR, Burns BJ and Borum R (2001). A randomized controlled trial of outpatient commitment in North Carolina. *Psychiatric Services*, 52, 325–9.

Tansella M and Thornicroft G (eds) (2001). *Mental Health Outcome Measures*. London: Gaskell.

Taylor R and Thornicroft R (2001). Uses and limits of randomised controlled trials in mental health service research. In *Mental Health Outcome Measures* M Tansella and G Thornicroft (eds). pp. 166–77. London: Gaskell.

Taylor SJ and Tweedie RL (1998a). A parametric 'trim and fill' method of assessing publication bias in meta-analysis: Department of Statistics, Colorado State University.

Taylor SJ and Tweedie RL (1998b). Trim and fill: a simple funnel plot based method of testing and adjusting for publication bias in meta-analysis: Department of Statistics, Colorado State University.

Teneback CC, Nahus Z and Speer AM (1999). Changes in prefrontal cortex and paralimbic activity in depression following two weeks of daily left prefrontal TMS. *Journal of Neuropsychiatry and Clinical Neuroscience*, 11, 426–35.

Thompson C, Kinmouth AL, Stevens L, Peveler RC, Stevens A, Ostler KJ, Pichering RM, Baker NG, Henson A, Preece J, Cooper D and Campbell MJ (2000). Effects of a clinical-practice guideline and practice-based education on detection and outcome of depression in primary care: Hampshire Depression Project randomised controlled trial. *Lancet*, 355, 185–91.

Thompson SG (1994). Why sources of heterogeneity in meta-analysis should be investigated. *British Medical Journal*, 309, 1351–5.

Thompson SG (1998). *Meta-analysis of clinical trials*, In Encyclopedia of Biostatistics, Volume 4, Armitage P and T Colton (eds), Wiley, Chichester.

Thompson SG and Higgins JPT (2002). How should meta-regression analyses be undertaken and interpreted? *Statistics in Medicine*, 21, 1559–76.

Thompson SG and Sharp SJ (1999). Exploring heterogeneity in meta-analysis: A comparison of methods. *Statistics in Medicine*, 18, 2693–708.

Thornley B and Adams C (1998). Content and quality of 2000 controlled trials in schizophrenia over 50 years. *British Medical Journal*, 317, 1181–4.

Tollefson G, Beasley C, Tran PV, Street JS, Krueger JA, Tamura RN, Graffeo KA and Thieme ME (1997). Olanzapine versus haloperidol in the treatment of schizophrenia and schizoaffective and schizophreniform disorders: results of an international collaborative trial. *American Journal of Psychiatry*, 154, 457–65.

Tollefson GD, Tran CB, Jr, Street JS, Krueger JA, Tamura N, Graffeo KA and Thieme ME (1997). Olanzapine versus haloperidol in the treatment of schizophrenia and schizoaffective and schizophreniform disorders: results of an international collaborative trial. *American Journal of Psychiatry*, 154, 457–65.

Truog RD, Randolph RWA and Morris A (1999). Is Informed Consent Always Necessary for Randomized, Controlled Trials? *New England Journal of Medicine*, 340, 804–7.

Tudor Hart J (1997). Response rates in South Wales, 1950–1996: changing requirements for mass participation in human research. In *Non-random Reflections on Health Services Research: On the 25th anniversary of Archie Cochrane's Effectiveness and Efficiency* (A Maynard and I Chalmers) (eds). London: BMJ Publishing Group.

UK 700 Group: Creed F, Burns T, Butler T, Byford S, Murray R, Thompson S and Tyrer P (1999). Comparison of intensive and standard case management for patients with psychosis. Rationale of the trial. *British Journal of Psychiatry*, 174, 74–8.

Urquhart J and de Klerk E (1998). Contending paradigms for the interpretation of data on patient compliance with therapeutic drug regimens. *Statistics in Medicine*, 17, 251–68.

Visser H (2001). Non-therapeutic research in the EU in adults incapable of giving consent, *Lancet*, 357, 818–19.

Wagner GS and Vankorff M (1995). Cost-effectiveness comparisons using 'real world' randomized trials: The case of new antidepressant drugs. *Journal of Clinical Epidemiology*, 48, 363–73.

Walker P and Klaassen MP (1995). Confidence intervals for cost-effectiveness ratio. *Health Economics*, 4, 373–81.

Walsh MM, Hilton JF, Masouredis CM, Gee L, Chesney MA and Ernster VL (1999). Smokeless tobacco cessation intervention for college athletes: Results after one year. *American Journal of Public Health*, 89, 228–34.

Ward E, King M, Lloyd M, Bower P, Sibbald B, Farrelly S, Gabbay M, Tarrier N and Addington-Hall J (2000). Randomized controlled trial on non-directive counselling, cognitive-behaviour therapy and usual general practitioner care for patients with depression I: clinical effectiveness. *British Medical Journal*, 321, 1383–8.

Warlow C (1990). How to do it. Organise a multicentre trial. *British Medical Journal*, 300, 180–3.

Waterhouse DM, Calzone KA, Mele C, *et al.* (1993). Adherence of oral tamoxifen: A comparison of patient self-report, pill count and microelectronic monitoring. *Journal of Clinical Oncology*, 11, 1189–97.

Watkins E, and Williams R (1998). The efficacy of cognitive-behavioural therapy *Cognitive Behavioural Therapy*, 8, 165–87.

Wentzer Licht R, Gouliqev G, Vestergaard PMF (1997). Generalisability of results from randomised drug trial : A trial on antimanic treatment *British Journal of Psychiatry*, 170, 264–7.

Wessely S, Bisson J and Rose S (2000). A systematic review of brief psychological interventions ("debriefing") for the treatment of immediate trauma related symptoms and the prevention of post traumatic stress disorder. In *Depression, Anxiety and Neurosis Module of the Cochrane Database of Systematic Reviews*, M Oakley-Browne, R Churchill, D Gill, *et al.* (eds). Oxford: Update Software.

Whitehead J (1986). Sample sizes for phase II and phase III clinical trials, in integrated approach. *Statistics in Medicine*, 5, 459–64.

Willian AR (2001). On the probability of cost-effectiveness using data from randomized clinical trials. *BMC Medical Research Methodology*, 1, 8.

Willian AR and Lin DY (2001). Incremental net benefit in randomized clinical trials. *Statistics in Medicine*, 20, 1563–74.

Willian AR, Lin DY, Cook RJ and Chen EB (2002). Using inverse-weighting in cost-effectiveness analysis with censored data. *Statistical Methods in Medical Research*, 11, 539–52.

Wittes S (2001). Randomized Treatment Assignment. In *Biostatistics in Clinical Trials*, C Redmond and T Colton (eds), pp. 384–92. Chichester: John Wiley.

Wood S, Ziedonis D, Sernyak M, Diaz E, Rosenheck R (2000). Characteristics of participants and non participants in medication trials for treatment of Schizophrenia, *Psychiatric Services*, 51, 79–84.

Yates F (1982). Regression models for repeated measurements. *Biometrics*, 38, 850–3.

Yusuf S, Willes J, Probstfield J and Tyroler HA (1991). Analysis and interpretation of treatment effects in subgroups of patients in randomized clinical trials. *Journal of the American Medical Association*, 266, 93–8.

Zeger SL and Liang KY (1986). Longitudinal data analysis for discrete and continuous outcomes. *Biometrics*, 42, 121–30.

Zelen M (1983). Guidelines for publishing papers on cancer clinical trials: responsibilities of editors and authors. *Journal of Clinical Oncology*, 1, 164–9.

Zimmerman M, Posternak M and Chelminski I (2002). Symptom severity and exclusion from antidepressant efficacy trials. *Journal of Clinical Psychopharmacology*, 22, 610–14.

Index